Imaging Dementia

Massimo Filippi • Federica Agosta

Imaging Dementia

Essentials for Clinical Practice

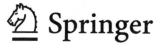 Springer

Massimo Filippi
Neuroimaging Research Unit
Division of Neuroscience
Neurology Unit
Neurorehabilitation Unit
Neurophysiology Service
IRCCS San Raffaele Scientific Institute
Milan
Italy

Vita-Salute San Raffaele University
Milan
Italy

Federica Agosta
Neuroimaging Research Unit
Neurology Unit
IRCCS San Raffaele Scientific Institute
Milan
Italy

Vita-Salute San Raffaele University
Milan
Italy

ISBN 978-3-030-66775-7   ISBN 978-3-030-66773-3   (eBook)
https://doi.org/10.1007/978-3-030-66773-3

This Springer imprint is published by the registered company Springer Nature Switzerland AG
The registered company address is: Gewerbestrasse 11, 6330 Cham, Switzerland

Acknowledgments

The authors take this opportunity to acknowledge gratefully the major contribution given by Edoardo G. Spinelli, Pietro M. Scamarcia, Giordano Cecchetti, and Giulia Donzuso in discussing and revising the content of this book from their diverse perspectives and expertise.

The authors are also thankful to Raffaella Migliaccio (Neurology Department and Paris Brain Institut, Pitié-Salpêtrière Hospital, Paris, France), and Marie-Odile Habert, and Aurélie Kas (Department of Nuclear Medicine, Pitié-Salpêtrière Hospital, Paris, France), for sharing illustrative figures.

Nomenclature

Advanced neuroimaging This term refers to neuroimaging techniques, which rely on materials and/or image post-processing available only in specialized centers, such as, for example, diffusion tensor MRI, resting state functional MRI, or PET imaging using experimental **tracers.**

Amyloid PET This is a biomarker used to demonstrate in vivo the presence of amyloid plaques in the brain, one of the main features of AD pathology. PET radioligands currently approved for clinical use include ^{18}F-florbetapir, ^{18}F-florbetaben, and ^{18}F-flutemetamol [1].

Conventional neuroimaging This term refers to standard neuroimaging techniques that are commonly used in a clinical context, either for the assessment of structural (i.e., compute tomography [CT], morphologic magnetic resonance imaging [MRI]) or functional (i.e., ^{18}F-Fluorodeoxyglucose Positron Emission Tomography [FDG-PET], dopamine transporter single-photon emission computed tomography [DaT-SPECT]) brain features.

Dementia Dementia, as defined in the Diagnostic and Statistical Manual of Mental Disorders-5 (DSM-5) [2], is an acquired condition marked by impairment in at least one cognitive domain that is severe enough to cause significant limitations in social and/or occupational functioning. Causes of dementia are categorized by their neuropathology, clinical features, and/or presumed etiology. The most common causes encountered in middle-aged and older individuals are Alzheimer's disease (AD), vascular, Lewy body, and frontotemporal dementia.

Diffusion-weighted (DW) MRI Diffusion-weighted (DW) MRI is a quantitative technique that exploits the diffusion of water within biological tissues [3]. The diffusion coefficient measures the ease of this translational motion of water. In biological tissues, this coefficient is lower than that in free water because the various structures of tissues (membranes, macromolecules, etc.) impede the free movement of water molecules. For this reason, the measured diffusion coefficient in biological systems is referred to as the "apparent diffusion coefficient" or ADC [3].

Diffusion tensor (DT) MRI Because some cellular structures (e.g., axons) impede movement to a greater degree in some directions than others (e.g., across as opposed to along the axon cylinder), the measured ADC also depends upon the direction in which the diffusion is measured. A full characterization of diffusion can be provided by the so-called tensor, which is a 3×3 matrix that characterizes the measured diffusion in three orthogonal directions [4]. From the diffusion tensor (DT) matrix, two scalar measures are derived. The first is the mean diffusivity (MD), which reflects the average diffusion in all three directions. The other measure, the fractional anisotropy (FA), measures the extent to which diffusion is nonuniform in the three orthogonal directions. DT MRI is typically used to assess the integrity of white matter tracts, as alterations of its parameters suggest axonal pathology and loss of structural connectivity within the brain [4].

Dopamine transporter (DaT) scan This term indicates single-photon emission computed tomography (SPECT) measurement of the striatal uptake of [^{123}I]ioflupane (or FP-CIT), a dopamine transporter (DaT) radioligand. It reflects the integrity of terminal fields of nigrostriatal neurons [5]. Loss of striatal DaT occurs in parkinsonian syndromes [5].

FDG-PET The most common radioligand used to assess brain function in PET studies is 2-[fluorine-28]fluoro-2-deoxy-D-glucose (FDG) [6], which is an analog of glucose, the main energy substrate of the brain. FDG, after uptake, is trapped within metabolically active cells so that signal emission mostly depends on cell metabolic activity. Synaptic dysfunction or loss, which is a main feature of brain damage and dementia, will induce a reduction in cell metabolism and energy demand, which is detected by FDG-PET studies.

Gray matter atrophy assessment T1-weighted MRI sequences are widely used to investigate alterations of gray matter structure, as they allow to visually assess and measure the overall brain volume, the pattern and rate of atrophy, and the volumes of specific regions of interest. Several post-processing analytical techniques can be applied to T1-weighted imaging, providing semi-automated measurements of gray matter volume loss at the voxel level (e.g., voxel-based morphometry) or cortical thinning.

Mild cognitive impairment (MCI) The term refers to the predementia symptomatic phase. In this phase, the cognitive impairment is both neither normal for age nor severe enough to affect subject's independence in functional abilities [7]. Affected cognitive domain is typically memory, and also language, executive, or other functions show an initial impairment.

Resting state functional MRI (RS fMRI) fMRI is able to measure brain activity by detecting changes associated with blood flow, based on the assumptions that cerebral blood flow and neuronal activation are coupled, and brain regions that are co-activated establish networks fundamental to maintain normal brain function [8]. The analysis of synchronous low-frequency (<0.1 Hz) fluctuations seen on fMRI scans at rest (i.e., in the absence of external stimulations) has demonstrated the presence of so-called resting-state networks of the human brain, which display synchronous variations of the blood-oxygenated-level-dependent signal. Assessing variations in the activity of resting state networks has provided important pathophysiological insights in normal aging [9] and several neurological conditions [10].

Subjective cognitive decline (SCD) SCD is defined as self-perceived cognitive decline among cognitively normal individuals. Some studies have suggested that SCD may be associated with an increased risk of incident MCI or dementia [11].

References

1. Villemagne VL, Dore V, Bourgeat P, et al. Abeta-amyloid and tau imaging in dementia. Semin Nucl Med. 2017;47:75–88.
2. American Psychiatric Association. Diagnostic and statistical manual of mental disorders. Washington, DC: American Psychiatric Association; 2013.
3. Le Bihan D, Mangin JF, Poupon C, et al. Diffusion tensor imaging: concepts and applications. J Magn Reson Imaging. 2001;13:534–46.
4. Basser PJ, Mattiello J, LeBihan D. Estimation of the effective self-diffusion tensor from the NMR spin echo. J Magn Reson B. 1994;103:247–54.

5. Brooks DJ, Ibanez V, Sawle GV, et al. Differing patterns of striatal 18F-dopa uptake in Parkinson's disease, multiple system atrophy, and progressive supranuclear palsy. Ann Neurol. 1990;28:547–55.
6. Ishii K. Clinical application of positron emission tomography for diagnosis of dementia. Ann Nucl Med. 2002;16:515–25.
7. Albert MS, DeKosky ST, Dickson D, et al. The diagnosis of mild cognitive impairment due to Alzheimer's disease: recommendations from the National Institute on Aging-Alzheimer's Association workgroups on diagnostic guidelines for Alzheimer's disease. Alzheimers Dement. 2011;7:270–9.
8. Logothetis NK. What we can do and what we cannot do with fMRI. Nature. 2008;453:869–78.
9. Damoiseaux JS, Beckmann CF, Arigita EJ, et al. Reduced resting-state brain activity in the "default network" in normal aging. Cereb Cortex. 2008;18:1856–64.
10. Greicius MD, Srivastava G, Reiss AL, Menon V. Default-mode network activity distinguishes Alzheimer's disease from healthy aging: evidence from functional MRI. Proc Natl Acad Sci U S A. 2004;101:4637–42.
11. van Harten AC, Mielke MM, Swenson-Dravis DM, et al. Subjective cognitive decline and risk of MCI: the Mayo clinic study of aging. Neurology. 2018;91:e300–12.

Introduction

Dementia is a syndrome characterized by the development of multiple cognitive deficits and behavioral changes that lead to impairment of functional activities. Dementia is a common condition in the elderly, especially the very elderly, and the absolute number of cases will continue to grow as the population ages. Every patient with cognitive decline deserves an assessment. There are potentially reversible conditions that may cause or mimic dementia, including brain tumors, normal pressure hydrocephalus, metabolic changes, infections, thyroid dysfunction, nutritional deficiencies (vitamin B_{12} being the most common), and dysimmune disorders (Table 1). Toxins, including chronic alcohol abuse, drugs or medication, may cause confusion and cognitive decline (Table 1). Sleep disorders and psychiatric diseases, such as depression, can be associated with cognitive deficits (Table 1). If detected and treated early, these cognitive problems can be reversed or their progress halted. However, the majority of cases of dementia are associated with primary degenerative, progressive, and irreversible diseases. An early accurate diagnosis of irreversible dementia is essential, too, to allow the disease to be tackled with available or experimental intervention, lifestyle changes, or logistical arrangements, before disability develops.

In the early and differential diagnosis of diseases leading to irreversible dementia, clinical history, which needs to be supplemented by an informant, should focus on the affected cognitive domains, the course of the illness, the impact on activity of daily living, and any associated noncognitive symptoms. Past medical history, comorbidities, family and education history are all important. A general and neurological physical examination should be performed in all patients. Neuropsychological assessment is central to diagnosis and management of disorders associated with cognitive impairment and should be performed, preferably, at an early stage of the disease. Laboratory tests should be used to explore whether the patient has comorbidity, risk factors for cognitive decline, or has a treatable cause for dementia (Table 1). Following clinical, neuropsychological, and laboratory evaluation, the diagnosis of irreversible dementias can be improved by the use of biological measures. Biomarkers of functional impairment, neuronal loss, and protein deposition that can be assessed by neuroimaging (i.e., magnetic resonance imaging [MRI] and positron emission tomography [PET]) or cerebrospinal fluid analysis are increasingly being used to diagnose Alzheimer's disease (AD) and other neurodegenerative

Table 1 Treatable causes of cognitive impairment and dementia

Etiology		Main features	Treatment	Typical neuroimaging findings
Toxic disorders	Drugs	Mainly due to drugs with anticholinergic properties, in elderly patients and during polipharmacotherapy (antihistamines, tricyclic antidepressants, antipsychotics, antimuscarinics)	Drug discontinuation	None
	Alcohol abuse	Anterograde and retrograde memory, apathy, intact sensorium, and relative preservation of long-term memory and other cognitive skills	Alcohol cessation	CT and MRI: enlargement of cerebral ventricles and sulci
Vitamin deficiencies	B_{12}	Most frequent, due to malabsorption of decreased intake. Associated with macrocytic anemia and neuropathy	Deficit correction	Not typical
	Folate	Associated with macrocytic anemia	Deficit correction	Not typical
	B_6	Associated with normocytic anemia, angular cheilitis, and glossitis	Deficit correction	Not typical
	B_1	Wernicke-Korsakoff syndrome: ataxia and ophthalmoplegia associated with confusion with acute onset. Related to alcohol abuse	Deficit correction	MRI—T2-weighted/FLAIR: symmetrically increased signal intensity in the mammillary bodies, dorsomedial thalami, tectal plate, periaqueductal gray matter, around the third ventricle MRI—T1-weighted (Gd): contrast enhancement can be seen in the same regions, most commonly the mammillary bodies

Endocrine disorders	Thyroid diseases	Hyper- and hypothyroidism	Hormone replacement/ antithyroid agents	Not typical
Structural disorders	Tumors	Both benign or malignant tumors, primitive or secondary	Surgery, radiotherapy, chemotherapy	CT and MRI—T1-weighted, T2-weighted, FLAIR: mass with altered signal with different features according to the tumor type; enhancement in T1-weighted with Gd
	Normal pressure hydrocephalus	Hakim's clinical triad: 1. Urinary incontinence 2. Deterioration in cognition (dementia) 3. Gait disturbances	Ventriculo-peritoneal shunt	• Marked dilatation of ventricles • Wide appearance of Sylvian and parasagittal CSF fissures • Wide aqueduct with a significant signal void in it from high-speed flow on MRI T2-weighted images • Lack of downward bending of the third ventricle floor • Periventricular edema • Narrow callosal angle of less than 90° • Increased Evans' ratio, more than 0.3
	Chronic subdural hematoma	Cognitive impairment, apathy, somnolence, and occasionally seizures	Neurosurgery	CT hypodensity and MRI hyperintensity— FLAIR is the most sensitive sequence
Infections	HIV	• Direct consequence of the HIV virus • Opportunistic infections • Neoplasm • Treatment-related complications	Anti-retroviral therapy, antimicrobic therapy, drug therapy monitoring	• Symmetric periventricular and deep white matter T2 hyperintensity on MRI • Confluent or patchy • No mass effect • No contrast enhancement
	Syphilis	Dementia with marked personality changes and tabes dorsalis	Antimicrobic therapy	Leptomeningeal enhancement, cerebral vasculitis, ischemic stroke, cerebral atrophy, and spinal cord atrophy

(continued)

Table 1 (continued)

Etiology		Main features	Treatment	Typical neuroimaging findings
Dysimmune disorders	Autoimmune encephalitis	Acute onset of cognitive deficits, seizures, acute onset of psychiatric disorders, dyskinesia (mainly in the face district)	High-dose steroids, intravenous immunoglobulin, plasma exchange	CT: negative MRI inconsistent findings: T2-FLAIR hyperintense demyelinating areas and Gd + areas in different regions. MRI often negative
	Paraneoplastic encephalitis	Acute onset of cognitive deficits, seizures, acute onset of psychiatric disorders	Treatment of the primitive tumor May be useful: high-dose steroids, intravenous immunoglobulin, plasma exchange	CT: negative MRI inconsistent findings: T2/FLAIR hyperintense demyelinating areas and Gd + areas in different regions. MRI often negative
Sleep disorders	Obstructive sleep apnea syndrome	Daytime sleepiness, memory and attention impairment, frequently associated with obesity and snoring	Continuous positive airway pressure, surgery	Not typical
Psychiatric disorders	Depression	Pseudodementia and associated cognitive dysfunction can be reversible	Antidepressants, psychotherapy	Not typical

Abbreviations: *CSF* cerebrospinal fluid, *CT* computed tomography, *FLAIR* fluid attenuated inversion recovery, *Gd* gadolinium (contrast agent), *HIV* human immunodeficiency virus, *MRI* magnetic resonance imaging

diseases in research studies and specialist clinical settings. However, the practical value of various neuroimaging techniques in clinical routine practice is not well defined yet and their potential future development is not fully appreciated.

The aim of this book is to guide the physicians in the choice of the available neuroimaging tools for a correct and cost-saving diagnosis and management of common primary, irreversible dementias. The book, which is concise in its content but profuse in its illustrative, tabular, and clinical case material, wishes to provide some practical and useful algorithms and rules to be used in the clinical setting.

AD is the most prevalent form of dementia: it accounts for 60% of cases of progressive cognitive impairment in aged individuals, age being the single most important risk factor. Thus, it is fitting that a chapter on an update on neuroimaging in AD kicks off this book. Chapter 2 is on vascular cognitive impairment (VCI), which is the second most common form of dementia after AD in terms of incidence and prevalence. Even though VCI is a common disorder, the diagnosis of pure vascular dementia is uncommon. Vascular pathology alone causes less than 10% of dementia cases, while it is an important contributive factor in multiple-etiology (also termed "mixed") dementia, mainly associated with AD pathology, accounting for approximately 30–40% of all dementia cases.

Chapter 3 of the book is focused on frontotemporal lobar degeneration (FTLD)—a devastating, relentlessly progressive, young onset, neurodegenerative disorder. FTLD typically shows a relatively focal and progressive atrophy involving the frontal or temporal lobes, or both. FTLD is less common than AD, with estimates of population prevalence ranging from 4 to 22 per 100,000 before age 65 years in Europe and the USA. However, this disease group is of incommensurate importance as a cause of young onset dementia and/or motor deficits, with all the global societal economic costs that this implies. Only in the past few decades has the clinical and pathological complexity of these diseases as paradigm of selective brain degeneration been fully appreciated.

In recent years we have increasingly recognized that Parkinson's disease (PD) and other parkinsonian syndromes do not simply feature disturbance of the motor function. Rather, patients with PD and other parkinsonisms also experience a multitude of non-motor symptoms commonly including cognitive impairment. Non-motor symptoms become increasingly prevalent over the course of the illness and are a major determinant of impaired quality of life and progression of disability.

In a later chapter, rapidly progressive dementias (RPD) are discussed. In contrast to most dementing conditions that take years to progress to death, RPD can be quickly fatal. It is critical to evaluate the RPD patient without delay to identify some peculiar features of specific diseases, as well as to rule out several treatable etiologies (i.e., tumors, autoimmune disorders). The chapter will discuss the general diagnostic workup of RPD, focusing on neuroimaging findings in prion diseases, which represents the main single etiology.

Dementia is becoming a major challenge for global health and social care. Neuroimaging is now considered as standard-of-care in the initial clinical assessment of patients with dementia. We hope that this book will be of practical relevance and assistance to practicing neurologists and radiologists in their daily activity and will also be an educational framework for trainees and researchers.

Contents

Alzheimer's Disease

1

Contents

1.1   Clinicopathological Findings

Alzheimer's disease (AD) is a progressive neurodegenerative disorder, irreversible and disabling, manifested by cognitive decline in different neuropsychological domains, progressive impairment in activities of daily living, and a variety of neuropsychiatric symptoms.

© Springer Nature Switzerland AG 2021
M. Filippi, F. Agosta, *Imaging Dementia*,
https://doi.org/10.1007/978-3-030-66773-3_1

1.1.1 Epidemiology and Risk Factors

AD is the most common cause of dementia in the elderly, accounting for up to 70–75% of all dementia cases [1, 2]. Its prevalence doubles every 5 years after age 65, ranging from approximately 2–3% in those 65–69 to 30% among individuals over 80. Moreover, the prevalence is higher in women than in men; in the age group 65–69 years, 0.7% of women and 0.6% of men suffer from the disease with increasing frequencies of 14.2% and 8.8% in individuals aged 85–89 years [3, 4].

Observational studies have identified several risk factors for AD, mostly overlapping cardiovascular ones (diabetes mellitus, smoking, depression, mental inactivity, physical inactivity, poor diet, etc.) [5] and explaining up to one-third of cases [6]. Different genetic factors have also been identified as increasing sporadic AD risk. The allele ε4 of the Apolipoprotein E (APOE) gene is the single genetic biggest risk factor for sporadic AD. Compared to non-ε4 carriers, ε4 heterozygotes have an odds ratio for AD of 3, rising to 12 in homozygotes [7]. Mutations in three genes (amyloid precursor protein-APP, presenilin 1-PSEN1, and presenilin 2-PSEN2) cause a rare (<0.5%) familial autosomal dominant form of AD [8].

1.1.2 Etiology and Pathophysiology

The cardinal features of AD pathology are diffuse extracellular amyloid-β (Aβ42) plaques and intracellular neurofibrillary tangles (NFTs), which are primarily composed of paired helical filaments of hyperphosphorylated tau (pTau) [9, 10]. The neuropathological processes underlying AD are associated with progressive neural and synapse loss, and then to macroscopic atrophy. According to amyloid hypothesis, an imbalance between Aβ production and Aβ clearance would lead to plaque formation. NFTs and subsequent neural dysfunction and degeneration are thought to be downstream processes [11]. Furthermore, awareness has grown about the existence of multiple pathological substrates associated with the AD clinical syndrome in the aged population. Mixed pathology is indeed frequently observed and includes vascular disease and dementia with Lewy bodies (DLB) pathology, even in familial AD [12, 13]. Recently, also limbic-predominant age-related TDP-43 encephalopathy (LATE) has been recognized as an important contributor to late-onset amnestic clinical syndromes of the AD type. In LATE, neuropathological examinations reveal cytoplasmic inclusions of phosphorylated TDP-43 protein associated to hippocampal neuron loss and gliosis, leading to hippocampal sclerosis [14].

1.1.3 Clinical Picture: The AD Continuum

Early clinical manifestations of AD may be either cognitive or neurobehavioral (e.g., depression, anxiety, and apathy). The typical and most common presentation of AD is of an elderly individual (i.e., >65 years old) with insidious, progressive problems of episodic memory (i.e., the ability to learn and retain new information) alone or in combination with the involvement of other cognitive domains. Typically, at this stage, a preservation of independence in functional abilities can be observed, defining thus the amnestic Mild Cognitive Impairment (MCI) status [15]. As the condition progresses, cognitive difficulties become more profound and widespread, affecting the other cognitive domains and finally interfering with activities of daily living [16]. At this stage, a diagnosis of dementia can be made. It has been estimated that 50% of MCI patients convert to dementia with rates of conversion at 5–10% per year [17, 18]. More recently, growing interest has been focused on subjective cognitive (memory) decline (SCD), a definition which refers to a personal experience of decreased cognitive function without objective signs of cognitive impairment from neuropsychological tests or daily functioning abilities [19]. Identifying those individuals who will progress to MCI and AD dementia is thought an unmet challenge.

More rarely, AD pathology subtends other clinical presentations that are encompassed under the general definition of "atypical AD syndromes" and are typically characterized by an earlier age at onset (i.e., <65 years) and a general preservation of short-term memory in the initial stages of the disease:

- Posterior cortical atrophy (PCA): characterized by insidious onset of predominant visual and praxis deficits, expression of occipital and parietal dysfunction [20, 21].
- Logopenic variant of primary progressive aphasia (lvPPA): characterized by prolonged word-finding pauses and impaired phonological short-term memory. Consistently, neuroimaging studies report asymmetric involvement of the temporoparietal junction of the dominant hemisphere [22].
- Frontal variant of AD: presenting chiefly with impairments of behavior and executive functions [23]. Frontal lobe involvement at neuroimaging studies is usually more prominent [24].

1.1.4   Diagnostic Criteria and Diagnostic Algorithm

A progressive change in cognition typically affecting memory is required to reinforce the diagnosis of a neurodegenerative disorder of the AD type. Preservation of independence in functional abilities is fundamental for a diagnosis of MCI due to AD [25]; alternatively, the patient is diagnosed with dementia [26].

Although the diagnosis remains essentially clinical, biomarkers are incorporated to strengthen the likelihood of subtending AD pathology. According to the 2011 NIA-AA MCI and AD Diagnostic Criteria [25–28], two classes of biomarkers are identified, one assessing the presence of brain amyloidopathy (identified by the letter "A"—low cerebrospinal fluid [CSF] Aβ42 and positive positron emission tomography [PET] amyloid imaging), and one mirroring neural degeneration (identified by the letter "N"—elevated CSF total Tau [tTau] and pTau, hypometabolism at PET with ^{18}F-fluorodeoxyglucose [FDG-PET] or atrophy on structural magnetic resonance imaging [MRI] in temporoparietal cortex). Regardless of whether clinical criteria for AD are fulfilled, when both A and N biomarkers are negative, the dementia is unlikely to be due to AD pathology.

Through the years, the need for an early diagnosis and implementation of reliable in vivo biomarkers, combined with the not optimum accuracy of pure clinical diagnosis (estimated sensitivity of 81% and specificity of 70% [29]), led progressively to defining AD as an exclusively biological construct, codified by biomarker combination and unlinked from its clinical expression. The new biomarker scheme proposed in 2018 by the NIA-AA committee [30, 31], labeled as A/T/N, implements a third class of biomarkers. In addition to those characterizing amyloid deposition (A) and neurodegeneration (N), indeed, a tauopathy biomarkers class (T) was recognized. The latter includes pTau pathology markers (CSF-pTau and Tau PET), whereas tTau keeps its role of aspecific neurodegeneration biomarker. Binarizing the aforementioned biomarkers, eight different "profiles" can be defined (Table 1.1), which can be grouped into three general "categories" based on biomarker profiles: normal A/T/N biomarkers; negative A but positive T and/or N (labeled "suspected non-Alzheimer's pathophysiology"); and those who are in the Alzheimer's continuum (positive A, regardless of T and N). To make a diagnosis of AD, a combination of positive A and T is needed.

In the clinical setting, a careful collection of past medical history and a complete clinical/neuropsychological assessment are clearly crucial for the evaluation of the type and entity of cognitive impairment. The cognitive stage of a subject (i.e., cognitively unimpaired, MCI, dementia) can be then combined with her/his biomarker

Table 1.1 Biomarkers profile and categories

AT(N) profiles	Biomarker category	
A− T− (N)−	Normal AD biomarkers	
A+ T− (N)−	Alzheimer pathologic change	*Alzheimer's continuum*
A+ T+ (N)−	AD	
A+ T+ (N)+	AD	
A+ T− (N)+	Alzheimer's and concomitant suspected non-Alzheimer's pathologic change	
A− T+ (N)−	Non-AD pathologic change	
A− T− (N)+	Non-AD pathologic change	
A− T+ (N)+	Non-AD pathologic change	

Reproduced with permission from Jack CR, Jr., Bennett DA, Blennow K, et al. NIA-AA Research Framework: Toward a biological definition of Alzheimer's disease. Alzheimers Dement 2018; 14:535–562, an open access article under the CC BY-NC-ND license
Abbreviations: *A* amyloidopathy biomarkers, *AD* Alzheimer's disease, *MCI* mild cognitive impairment, *N* neurodegeneration biomarkers, *T* tauopathy biomarkers

Table 1.2 Biomarker profile and cognitive stage

Syndromal cognitive stage

		Cognitively unimpaired	MCI	Dementia
Biomarker profile	A− T− (N)−	Normal AD biomarkers and cognitively unimpaired	Normal AD biomarkers with MCI	Normal AD biomarkers with dementia
	A+ T− (N)−	Preclinical Alzheimer's pathologic change	Alzheimer's pathologic change with MCI	Alzheimer's pathologic change with dementia
	A+ T− (N)+	Alzheimer's and concomitant suspected non-Alzheimer's pathologic change, cognitively unimpaired	Alzheimer's and concomitant suspected non-Alzheimer's pathologic change with MCI	Alzheimer's and concomitant suspected non-Alzheimer's pathologic change with dementia
	A+ T+ (N)−	Preclinical Alzheimer's disease	Alzheimer's disease with MCI (prodromal AD)	Alzheimer's disease with dementia
	A+ T+ (N)+			

Reproduced with permission from Jack CR, Jr., Bennett DA, Blennow K, et al. NIA-AA Research Framework: Toward a biological definition of Alzheimer's disease. Alzheimers Dement 2018; 14:535–562, an open access article under the CC BY-NC-ND license
Abbreviations: *A* amyloidopathy biomarkers, *AD* Alzheimer's disease, *MCI* mild cognitive impairment, *N* neurodegeneration biomarkers, *T* tauopathy biomarkers

profile, as shown by Table 1.2. It must be underlined how for a given cognitive stage, different biomarkers profiles could be present in the population. Likewise, different cognitive stages may be present for the same biomarker profile [31].

Core diagnostic criteria of PCA [20, 21] comprise a gradual and prominent early disturbance of visual and other posterior cognitive functions (e.g., oculomotor apraxia, optic ataxia, acalculia, limb apraxia, and simultanagnosia). Anterograde memory and executive functions are relatively spared in the early phases, and a predominant occipital-parietal or occipito-temporal involvement is recognized at both structural (MRI) and metabolic (PET) brain imaging techniques.

The diagnosis of lvPPA requires that both core clinical criteria [22] are present at the same time (impaired single-word retrieval and repetition of sentences and phrases) in addition to at least three of the four additional features (phonologic errors, spared single-word comprehension and object knowledge, spared motor speech, absence of agrammatism). Both structural (MRI) and metabolic (PET) brain imaging show the involvement of the left temporoparietal junction.

In frontal variant of AD, a prominent initial behavioral and/or dysexecutive impairment can be recognized, which makes the distinction from frontotemporal lobar degeneration (FTLD) challenging. An initial additional impairment in episodic memory and a predominant atrophy of temporoparietal lobes at MRI evaluation, though, help discriminate the frontal variant of AD from FTLD [24].

Furthermore, an aged person presenting with an amnestic syndrome of the Alzheimer type, combined with N biomarkers suggestive for medial temporal involvement and negative A and/or T biomarkers, could reasonably pertain to LATE neuropathological change [14].

After an agreement achieved among interdisciplinary experts in the field, weighting the specific utility of the individual biomarkers based on available evidence and clinical expertise, a theoretical diagnostic algorithm has been recently proposed suggesting the optimal timepoint for neuroimaging biomarkers for early and differential diagnosis of AD and other neurodegenerative diseases that can lead to dementia (Fig. 1.1) [32]. Three main diagnostic pathways with distinct biomarker sequences depending on the clinical presentation were proposed. According to this diagnostic workup [32], the clinical/neuropsychological evaluation should be followed by structural imaging when needed to establish reliable etiological diagnosis (Fig. 1.1). Further workup could be halted, if clinical and structural imaging information both converge toward a specific diagnosis, e.g., in patients with memory predominant profile with typical hippocampal atrophy, possibly with positive family history and/or ε4-positive APOE genotype when available, and/or if consequences of the diagnosis are poor (e.g., other comorbidities dominating patient prognosis). However, if tailored therapy concepts are the aim and/or decisions depend on a conclusive diagnosis and prognosis, additional biomarker assessment is required. In *pathway 1*, preferred if the main suspicion is AD, analysis of amyloid pathology using PET or CSF would be the subsequent next step (Fig. 1.1). Depending on the result, FDG-PET may be additionally required to obtain further prognostic/diagnostic information, e.g., on the extent of neurodegeneration or on a specific pattern of hypometabolism or with regard to short-term prognosis in MCI (Fig. 1.1). *Pathway 2* is recommended if AD is not the single most probable/suspected diagnosis or for older (>75–80 years) individuals. If the result of the FDG-PET scan is conclusive (see other chapters for further details), no further test might be requested; in contrast, if the pattern of FDG-PET hypometabolism is not conclusive, or if the reliable clarification of neuropathology is clinically relevant, a further amyloid test (PET or CSF) might be necessary (Fig. 1.1). Finally, in *Pathway 3*, a dopamine transporter single-photon emission computed tomography (DaT-SPECT) (or I^{123}-meta-iodobenzylguanidine [mIBG] myocardial scintigraphy) would be recommended as the primary test for all situations in which a movement disorder/parkinsonian syndrome is clinically in question; in some cases (abnormal DaT-SPECT), no further test is required, but if further specification is needed (i.e., if the DaT-SPECT is normal, or, if it is abnormal, to differentiate between all neurodegenerative parkinsonian syndrome), then an additional FDG-PET is recommended, followed by amyloid PET if AD remains a possibility (see Chap. 4 for further details).

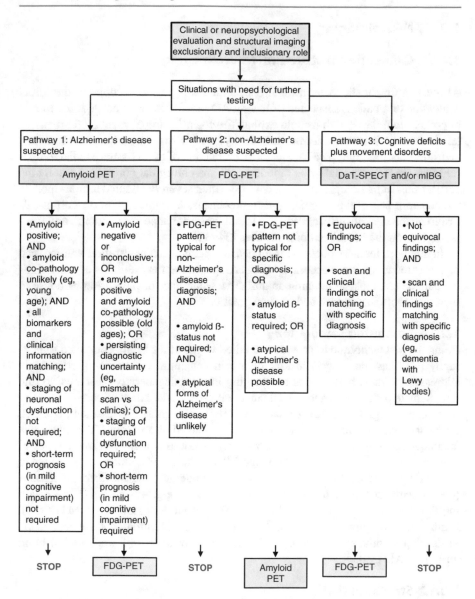

Fig. 1.1 Proposal for a diagnostic algorithm for early and differential diagnoses of dementia. The algorithm has been recently proposed to suggest the optimal timepoint for neuroimaging biomarkers for early and differential diagnosis of AD and other neurodegenerative diseases that can lead to dementia. It is a theoretical proposal and further validation of the order of tests is needed. See text for details. Abbreviations: *FDG-PET* ^{18}F-fluorodeoxyglucose positron emission tomography, *mIBG*[123]I-meta-iodobenzylguanidine imaging. (Reproduced with permission from Chételat GAJ, Barthel H, Garibotto V, et al. Amyloid-PET and ^{18}F-FDG-PET in the diagnostic investigation of Alzheimer's disease and other dementias. Lancet Neurol 2020; 19:951–962)

1.2   Neuroimaging

1.2.1   Conventional Structural Neuroimaging

All current diagnostic criteria require structural imaging to be done at the initial evaluation of a patient suspected of having AD [25–28]. This is needed first to rule out other brain diseases that could explain the cognitive impairment (cerebrovascular diseases, brain tumors, normal pressure hydrocephalus, etc.) (Fig. 1.1). Moreover, neurodegeneration in typical AD leads to a reduction of brain tissue. Medial temporal lobes (MTL), especially the hippocampus and entorhinal cortex, are among the earliest sites of pathologic involvement [33]. Other severely affected regions include the posterior part of the cingulate gyrus, precuneus, and splenium of the corpus callosum on the medial surface, and the parietal, posterior superior temporal, and frontal regions on the lateral cerebral surfaces [34–36].

In addition, features obtained from neuroimaging, such as cerebral volume, can be measured much more accurately than changes in memory abilities or other clinical parameters, making imaging an attractive technique for measuring response to treatment, both in research and clinical practice.

1.2.1.1 Computed Tomography

Being the first technique to provide a detailed image of the brain, computed tomography (CT) has the longest history of use in dementia. CT scanning adequately addresses the most basic needs for imaging in neurodegenerative diseases; to rule out alternate pathologies and to evaluate the presence and extent of cerebrovascular disease. Although CT is still regularly used for the diagnostic assessment, research on most aspects of degenerative dementia has moved away from CT because this technique has lower resolution than MRI and is not as sensitive to many types of abnormalities seen in AD [37]. Although MRI is the favorite imaging technique in the workup of dementia, some patients cannot undergo MRI for different reasons (e.g., pacemaker and claustrophobia). In these cases, a high-resolution CT scan with multiplanar reconstruction can be used for visual assessment of MTL [38]. Furthermore, despite the lower contrast resolution of CT, attempts have been made to develop automated CT segmentation methods to detect and track global brain atrophy in AD [39].

1.2.1.2 Structural MRI

MRI is surely the first-choice neuroimaging technique in a patient with suspected AD, allowing the early identification of brain atrophy patterns related to AD pathology, even before measurable changes in memory [40]. The essential MR sequences that provide the important minimum set of information required to be addressed in a subject with suspected cognitive impairment due to AD are as follows:

- T1-weighted images with thin slices and multiplanar reconstruction to detect regional atrophy. In particular, coronal T1-weighted imaging should be acquired to assess MTL atrophy [41, 42].

- T2-weighted and fluid-attenuated inversion recovery (FLAIR) images to detect white matter alterations.
- Conventional T2*-weighted gradient recall-echo (GRE) or susceptibility-weighted imaging (SWI) to detect signal alterations derived from microbleeds. Both white matter hyperintensities and microbleeds could be indeed expression of cerebrovascular pathology (i.e., small vessel disease and/or cerebral amyloid angiopathy), often coexistent with AD (see Chap. 2 for further details) [43].

Regarding the field strength, the use of a 3T scanner might be preferred, but images of a modern 1.5T MRI scanner have also an acceptable definition and represent a good choice for the clinical use [44].

Of all the structural markers of AD, hippocampal atrophy assessed on coronal T1-weighted images is the best established and validated. MRI-autopsy studies have convincingly corroborated that hippocampal volumes measured from antemortem MRI scans correlate with Braak NFTs pathologic staging [45, 46]. Although MTL atrophy is proposed by the most recent research diagnostic criteria as a neurodegeneration biomarker, thus not specific for AD, it is still used in the clinical practice to support a diagnosis of AD (Fig. 1.2) [26, 31]. In particular, MTL volume can be estimated through procedures with variable levels of automation: (a) visual rating scales allow a categorization of MTL atrophy into discrete levels of increasing severity; (b) MTL structures can be manually labeled and volumes can be computed; (c) automated algorithms can refer an individual digital brain to a reference template on a voxel-by-voxel basis and subsequently identify and measure different brain structures [47].

Several visual rating scales to quantify the degree of MTL atrophy have been developed [48–51]. These scales have a high accuracy in determining the extent of atrophy in cross-sectional studies and reached an accuracy of about 89% in

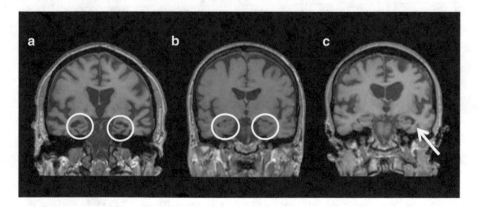

Fig. 1.2 (a) Coronal T1-weighted MRI showing symmetrical medial temporal lobe (MTL) atrophy in a patient with Alzheimer's disease (circled). (b) Coronal T1-weighted MRI showing relative sparing of MTL structures in dementia with Lewy bodies (circled). (c) Coronal T1-weighted MRI showing highly asymmetric left MTL atrophy (arrow) in frontotemporal lobar degeneration

discriminating AD patients from controls in a small sample of subjects [50]. In the past years, automated segmentation software to trace and quantify the volume of MTL structures has been developed, and support vector machine classifiers have been applied, reaching 82% sensitivity and 90% specificity in differentiating mild AD from healthy controls [52]. However, at present, accepted standards for quantitative analysis of hippocampal volumetry are lacking [53, 54]; indeed, although manual hippocampal segmentation is the most validated procedure to estimate hippocampal volume, different laboratories use different anatomical landmarks and measurement approaches [54]. The use of multivariate analysis and support vector machine classifier algorithms in combination with quantitative voxel-based methods might be the key to establish a disease model to be compared with each individual subject with a clinical suspect of AD.

In order to assess the specificity of structural MRI findings to indicate underlying AD pathology, several studies have also reported the relationship between hippocampal volumes and either cortical amyloid burden (amyloid PET scans) or CSF Aβ42 in cognitively unimpaired and MCI subjects [55–58]. This relationship was strongest in unimpaired patients in the inferior-anterior hippocampal head and superior and inferior hippocampal body, but in the MCI group the relationship was limited to the superior body. This could mean that this relation may decrease with disease progression. Moreover, studies focusing on atrophy rate, rather than cross-sectional ones, demonstrated a higher correlation to CSF Aβ42 in preclinical AD, while CSF pTau levels relate more to brain atrophy rates later in the disease progression [57, 59, 60].

Clinical population studies have reported that hippocampal volumes in mild AD patients are 15–40% smaller than controls [61, 62], and in MCI the volume is reduced by 10–15% [63]. MTL volumes can separate AD patients and MCI subjects from healthy controls, with accuracy ranging from 70% for early stages of MCI to complete group separation for advanced stages of AD dementia [61]. Furthermore, volumes of hippocampus and entorhinal cortex predict future conversion to AD in individuals with MCI with an accuracy of approximately 80–85%, with a slightly greater predictive value for the entorhinal cortex compared to the hippocampus [64–66]. A meta-analysis estimated that MTL volume, as assessed on structural MRI, has 73% sensitivity and 81% specificity for predicting whether patients with MCI will convert to AD [67].

Several studies report correlations between regional brain volume or atrophy and various types of cognitive tests. As expected, memory tests correlate with MTL volumes, while executive function typically correlate more strongly with whole brain atrophy [68–70]. In a recent longitudinal study on unimpaired subjects, among patients with baseline positive amyloid PET scans, the presence of MTL atrophy was associated to a more rapid decline in verbal memory, visual memory, and language tests [71].

As previously anticipated, atrophy in AD extends beyond MTL, including the medial and inferior temporal lobes, temporoparietal association neocortex, and frontal lobes (Fig. 1.3) [72–74]. Furthermore, all these areas are involved by early AD pathology [9]. Consistently, compared to MCI subjects who remain stable over

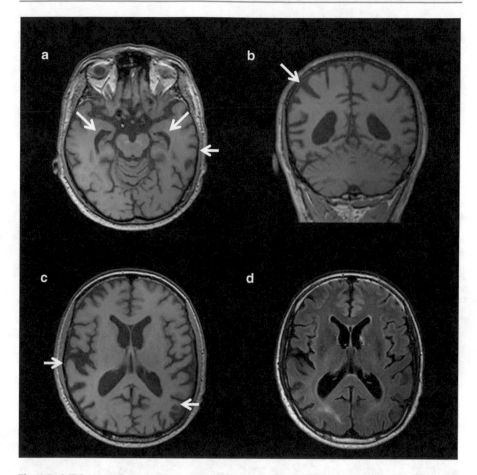

Fig. 1.3 MRI scans of a typical late-onset Alzheimer's disease (AD) presentation. Axial (**a, c**) and coronal (**b**) T1-weighted MR scans showing atrophy of the temporoparietal regions, including the hippocampi (arrows). FLAIR MR scan (**d**) shows white matter hyperintensities consistent with cerebrovascular disease, often coexistent with AD

time, MCI converters to AD have distinct patterns of gray matter atrophy, showing atrophy not only in MTL but also in the abovementioned areas [75].

Moreover, increasing interest has grown in SCD status, which is considered the prodromal phase of AD [19]. It has been shown that 14% of individuals with normal cognitive function and subjective cognitive decline develop dementia after 4 years followup [76]. MRI studies focusing on subjective memory decline population mainly found a decreased hippocampal volume when compared to cognitively unimpaired subjects; as for MCI, atrophy seems to extend beyond the hippocampus, involving also entorhinal cortex and amygdala, anterior cingulate, medial prefrontal cortex, cuneus, and precuneus [77–79].

When speaking of AD, a separate discussion must be done for early-onset presentation of the disease (EOAD; i.e., subjects showing onset of symptoms before the age of 65 years). In general, EOAD patients with amnestic presentation are characterized by a more widespread gray and white matter loss in the temporoparietal cortex than classic late-onset AD, characterized by more focal MTL involvement (Fig. 1.4a) [80–82]. Consistently, EOAD show a more rapid clinical course and greater impairment in all cognitive domains [81].

Differently from classical amnestic syndrome, in atypical AD presentations, the MTL is relatively spared [83, 84]. Despite this, a pattern of temporoparietal atrophy or cortical thinning may suggest AD pathology even in subjects presenting with

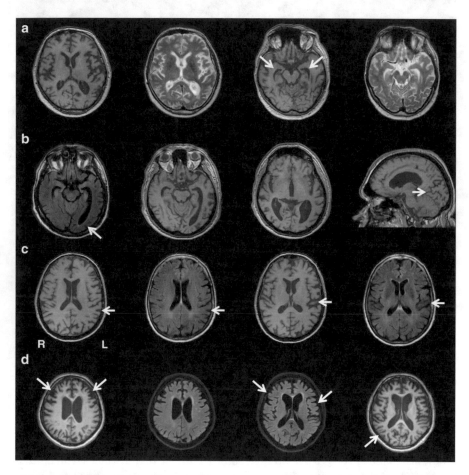

Fig. 1.4 MRI scans of early-onset Alzheimer's disease (AD) presentations. (**a**) Early-onset AD: T1- and T2-weighted axial MR scans showing a widespread atrophy of the frontal and temporoparietal regions, including the hippocampi (arrows). (**b**) Posterior cortical atrophy: FLAIR and T1-weighted axial MR images showing lateral temporal, parietal, and occipital atrophy, enlargement of posterior horns of lateral ventricles (arrow). T1-weighted sagittal MR image shows focal occipital sulci enlargement (arrow). (**c**) Logopenic variant of primary progressive aphasia: T1-weighted and FLAIR axial MR images showing atrophy of the left temporoparietal junction and inferior parietal lobule (arrows). (**d**) Frontal variant of AD: T1-weighted and FLAIR MR scans showing bilateral atrophy of frontal and parietal lobes (arrows). *L* left, *R* right

non-amnestic clinical syndromes [84, 85]. More specifically, structural MRI scans of patients with PCA show atrophy of parieto-occipital and posterior temporal cortices (Fig. 1.4b) [83, 86]. Compared with typical AD cases, PCA patients have greater parietal and less MTL atrophy [83]. In lvPPA, the pattern of atrophy primarily affects the left temporoparietal junction, including the left posterior superior and middle temporal gyri, as well as the inferior parietal lobule (Fig. 1.4c) [22, 83]. The involvement of the left MTL has been reported less consistently [22]. Such a posterior temporoparietal pattern of atrophy may help discriminating this syndrome from the other subtypes of PPA. The frontal variant of AD typically shows greater involvement of various prefrontal and temporal regions than typical AD (Fig. 1.4d). Moreover, when compared with frontotemporal lobar degeneration (FTLD) patients, frontal AD subjects show a greater involvement of posterior brain regions (Fig. 1.4d) (see Chap. 3 for further details) [24].

Beside atrophy, cerebrovascular pathology has been associated with AD, especially in the late-onset form. White matter hyperintensities, lacunes, and microbleeds can be observed on T2-weighted and FLAIR MRI scans of AD patients. An overlap with vascular cognitive impairment (VCI) may occur, as patients may actually fulfill both criteria for AD and VCI (see Chap. 2 for further details).

1.2.2 Molecular Imaging

1.2.2.1 SPECT and FDG-PET

The nuclear medicine techniques most frequently used in the clinical assessment of AD and other neurodegenerative diseases are SPECT and FDG-PET [87]. SPECT and FDG-PET scans of typical AD patients demonstrate predominant hypoperfusion or reduced glucose metabolism of the temporoparietal regions, including the precuneus and posterior cingulate cortex (Fig. 1.5) [87]. SPECT is technically less demanding, while FDG-PET is more sensitive, mainly due to its higher resolution

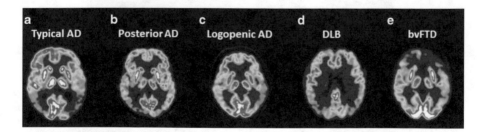

Fig. 1.5 FDG-PET patterns associated with typical late-onset Alzheimer's disease (AD) (**a**), atypical AD variants (**b**, posterior cortical atrophy; **c**, logopenic variant of primary progressive aphasia) compared with non-AD dementias (**d**, dementia with Lewy bodies; **e**, behavioral variant of frontotemporal dementia). *AD* Alzheimer's disease, *bvFTD* behavioral variant of frontotemporal dementia, *DLB* dementia with Lewy bodies. (Reprinted by permission from Springer Nature, European Journal of Nuclear Medicine, Clinical utility of FDG-PET for the differential diagnosis among the main forms of dementia, Nestor PJ, Altomare D, Festari C, et al. © 2018)

[88], but comes at the cost of more complex detector system and tracer production facilities. In general, the magnitude of hypometabolism seen with FDG-PET is greater than the amplitude of hypoperfusion seen with SPECT [88].

FDG-PET has been largely shown in the last decades to be a promising technique for detecting functional brain changes in AD, even in prodromal stages (Fig. 1.6). FDG-PET studies showed high diagnostic accuracy in AD (sensitivity ranging from 78% to 98% and specificity ranging from 78% to 98%) confirming its superior diagnostic accuracy over SPECT [89–91]. FDG-PET has been shown to be able to

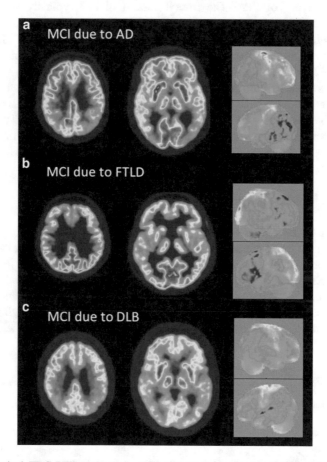

Fig. 1.6 Typical FDG-PET patterns in mild cognitive impairment (MCI). (**a**) MCI due to Alzheimer's disease (AD). Left parietal, precuneus, and posterior cingulate hypometabolism. (**b**) MCI due to frontotemporal lobar degeneration. Bilateral frontal hypometabolism (more marked in the left inferior frontal as shown in the 3D-Statistical Surface Projections [SSP] images) and striatum. (**c**) MCI due to dementia with Lewy bodies. Bilateral parieto-occipital hypometabolism, mainly left hemisphere with relative preservation in posterior cingulate cortex (cingulate island sign). *AD* Alzheimer's disease, *DLB* dementia with Lewy bodies, *FTLD* frontotemporal lobar degeneration, *MCI* mild cognitive impairment. (Reprinted by permission from Springer Nature, European Journal of Nuclear Medicine, Clinical utility of FDG-PET for the clinical diagnosis in MCI, Arbizu J, Festari C, Altomare D, et al. © 2018)

differentiate patients with AD from subjects with DLB with 83% sensitivity and 85% specificity [92], and from patients with FTLD with 99% sensitivity and 98% (Fig. 1.5) [93–95]. A single-center cohort study of 44 subjects with variable levels of cognitive impairment and autopsy confirmation showed that the diagnostic accuracy of FDG-PET at an initial clinical evaluation (sensitivity, 84%; specificity, 74%) was better than that of initial clinical evaluation alone (sensitivity, 76%; specificity, 58%), and was similar to that of longitudinal clinical diagnosis over approximately 4 years [96]. The clinical diagnosis of AD was associated with a 70% probability of detecting AD pathology, but with a positive FDG-PET scan this increased to 84%; with a negative FDG-PET scan it decreased to 31% [96]. A diagnosis of not-AD at an initial clinical evaluation was associated with a 35% probability of AD pathology, increasing to 70% with a positive PET scan [96].

Multiple studies used FDG-PET in patients with MCI. In general, they show regional hypometabolism consistent with AD, even if typically limited to posterior cingulate cortex and MTL (Fig. 1.6) [95, 97–99]. Another important application of FDG-PET in the MCI evaluation is its ability to predict progression to dementia. Normal FDG uptake in MCI indicates a low chance of progression within 2 years, despite the presence of an amnestic disorder at neuropsychological testing [100]. On the contrary, basal positive FDG-PET scans were found to detect MCI patients who had converted into AD within 2 years with a sensitivity of 81% and a specificity of 97% [101]. The progression of AD is accompanied by a continued increase and spreading of hypometabolism [100, 102, 103]. Two studies including unimpaired and MCI subjects have shown greater hypometabolism rates in those with demonstrated amyloid pathology at baseline [104, 105].

Overall hypoperfusion or hypometabolism in EOAD is much greater in magnitude and extent than that of late-onset AD patients with similar dementia severity [106, 107]. Distinct hypometabolism patterns are also found in the main AD variants: left inferior frontal and left tempo-parietal in lvPPA (accuracy of 89% in differentiating lvPPA from typical AD) (Fig. 1.7), and bilateral

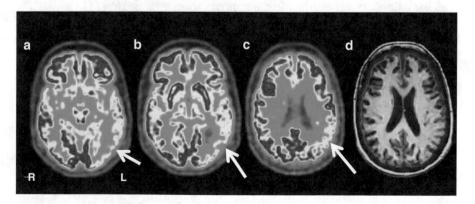

Fig. 1.7 (**a–c**) FDG-PET scan showing left-lateralized temporal and parietal hypometabolism (arrows) in a patient with logopenic variant of primary progressive aphasia, and (**d**) corresponding PET/MRI fusion image. *L* left, *R* right

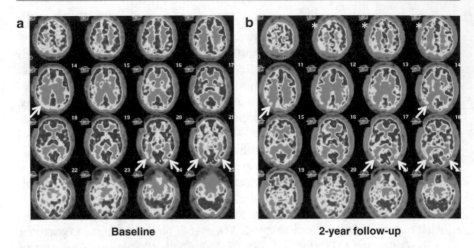

Baseline   **2-year follow-up**

Fig. 1.8 (**a**) ^{99m}Tc SPECT scan showing bilateral hypoperfusion of parietal and occipital cortical areas (arrows) in a patient with posterior cortical atrophy at first clinical evaluation, and (**b**) the same scan performed after 2 years of clinical follow-up, demonstrating worsening of the hypoperfusion in the same regions (arrows), as well as initial involvement of frontal areas (asterisks)

occipito-parieto-temporal in PCA (accuracy 91% in distinguishing PCA from typical AD) (Fig. 1.8) [108, 109]. In addition to posterior regions, FDG-PET in PCA typically show specific areas of hypometabolism in the frontal eye fields bilaterally (Fig. 1.8), which can occur secondary to the loss of input from occipitoparietal regions and be associated with oculomotor apraxia in these patients [110, 111]. Frontal variant of AD shows greater medial and orbital frontal hypometabolism than typical AD patients, likely reflecting a greater pathological load in these brain regions [112]. A retrospective study of 94 patients with a clinical diagnosis of MCI or dementia (typical or atypical), who had an FDG-PET within 2 months of their diagnosis, showed that FDG-PET findings significantly lowered the number of atypical/unclear diagnoses from 39% to 16% [113].

As for subjective cognitive decline forms, the European Association of Nuclear Medicine and European Academy of Neurology do not recommend the use of FDG-PET as critical outcomes were not available in any of the examined papers [94].

1.2.2.2 Amyloid Imaging

Amyloid radioligands typically bind to insoluble fibrillar forms of Aβ40 and Aβ42 deposits, which are a major component of neuritic plaques and vascular deposits. ^{11}C-labeled Pittsburgh Compound-B (^{11}C-PIB) was the first agent to be used in humans in 2002. Although it has demonstrated a very high sensitivity for AD (90% or greater), due to its short half-life (20 min), the use of ^{11}C-PIB PET has been limited to research centers [114]. Aβ tracers labeled with fluorine-18 (half-life up to 115 min) have subsequently been developed for clinical use, and in 2012 U.S. Food and Drug Administration approved the first Aβ imaging PET probe, ^{18}F-florpetabir [115]. Subsequently also ^{18}F-flutemetamol and ^{18}F-florbetaben have been approved

[116, 117]. All amyloid ligands have demonstrated an almost optimal sensitivity and specificity in detecting AD by visual interpretation [115, 117–120].

Amyloid tracer binding in AD patients is diffuse and symmetric, with high uptake consistently found in the prefrontal cortex, precuneus, and posterior cingulate cortex, followed by the lateral parietal, lateral temporal cortex, and striatum (Fig. 1.9). This pattern closely mirrors the distribution of plaques found at autopsy [121]. EOAD patients show increased ^{11}C-PIB uptake throughout frontal, parietal and lateral temporal cortices, and striatum, demonstrating in general higher radioligand uptake compared with late-onset AD [107, 122, 123]. Of particular interest is the potential of PET amyloid imaging to differentiate mixed AD with cerebrovascular disease from pure VCI [124], and AD from FTLD, which is not associated with amyloid deposition (Fig. 1.9) [125–127].

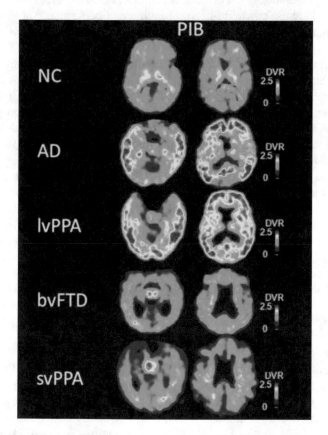

Fig. 1.9 Typical ^{11}C-labeled Pittsburgh Compound B (PIB) binding for normal controls, Alzheimer's disease, logopenic variant of primary progressive aphasia, behavioral variant of frontotemporal dementia, and semantic variant of primary progressive aphasia. *AD* Alzheimer's disease, *bvFTD* behavioral variant of frontotemporal dementia, *DVR* distribution volume ratio, *lvPPA* logopenic variant of primary progressive aphasia, *NC* normal controls, *svPPA* semantic variant of primary progressive aphasia. (Reprinted by permission from Springer Nature, Alzheimers Res Ther, Amyloid imaging in the differential diagnosis of dementia: review and potential clinical applications, Laforce R, Jr., Rabinovici GD. © 2011)

In MCI due to AD patients, ^{11}C-PIB uptake has been shown to be comparable to that seen in AD [128]. Additionally, it is predictive of progression to AD and the risk ranges from 50% to 80% compared to 0–10% in subjects with amyloid-negative imaging [129, 130].

There have been efforts to estimate the impact of amyloid PET in the clinical management of suspected AD patients. In one study, the authors assessed the impact of ^{18}F-florbetapir imaging in 229 patients, and reported a change in diagnosis in 54.6% of patients after PET scan with an increase in diagnostic confidence of 21.6% [131]. A negative amyloid PET scan reduces the likelihood that cognitive impairment is due to AD, but a positive scan does not allow a diagnosis [132, 133]. Indeed, approximately 25–35% of cognitively unimpaired elderly subjects, as demonstrated by postmortem reports, show high cortical radioligand retention in the prefrontal, posterior cingulate cortex, and precuneus regions [115, 119, 120, 134]. Unlike AD, a correlation between amyloid imaging binding and performance at memory tests has been demonstrated in MCI and cognitively unimpaired subjects [115, 119, 120, 135].

In vivo studies using ^{11}C-PIB PET in patients with an atypical clinical presentation of AD have reported greater PIB uptake in occipital cortex in PCA [136–139], and left temporoparietal regions in PPA [136] in single cases or in small series studies. However, larger studies have found no difference in PIB retention patterns in PCA or PPA compared with amnestic AD [125, 140–142]. All showed diffuse ^{11}C-PIB uptake throughout frontal, temporoparietal, and occipital cortex, independent of the clinical presentation (Fig. 1.9).

According to the abovementioned theoretical diagnostic algorithm for AD that has been recently proposed (Fig. 1.1) [32], amyloid imaging is recommended after structural imaging has been performed and in case of atypical presentation, ambiguous structural imaging pattern, or in case the amyloid status has to be confirmed (e.g., for the administration of disease-modifying therapies). Likewise, amyloid PET is useful in case of suspected non-AD pathology in the absence of a disease-specific pattern of hypometabolism at FDG-PET. Furthermore, amyloid imaging is likely to find clinical utility for the stratification of MCI patients in which clinical uncertainty exists, and for the evaluation of patients with early-onset progressive cognitive decline.

1.2.2.3 Tau Imaging

Benzimidazole pyrimidine derivate ^{18}F-flortaucipir, also known as ^{18}F-AV-1451, exhibits high binding affinity to the paired helical filaments of pTau, and high binding selectivity for Tau over $A\beta$ in AD brains [143–145]. Additionally, postmortem analysis revealed that ^{18}F-flortaucipir binding correlates with postmortem NFTs Braak staging in AD brains [146, 147]. Longitudinal studies in AD patients have also demonstrated that the spatial patterns of tracer distribution follow the known distribution of NFTs [148].

Accuracy of ^{18}F-flortaucipir PET in differentiating MCI and AD patients from healthy subjects is 93% [149]. Moreover, selective tracer retention patterns can be found in AD patients presenting with a variety of clinical phenotypes [150]: patients

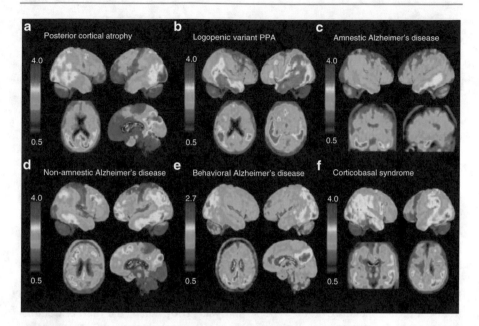

Fig. 1.10 Typical ^{18}F-AV1451 (flortaucipir) binding for patients with different presentations of the Alzheimer's disease (AD) continuum, including (**a**) posterior cortical atrophy, (**b**) logopenic variant of primary progressive aphasia, (**c**) typical amnestic AD, (**d**) non-amnestic AD, (**e**) behavioral/frontal AD, and (**f**) corticobasal syndrome with AD pathology. (Reproduced from Ossenkoppele R, Schonhaut DR, Scholl M, et al. Tau PET patterns mirror clinical and neuroanatomical variability in Alzheimer's disease. Brain 2016; 139:1551–1567, by permission of Oxford University Press)

with an amnestic presentation show highest ligand retention in MTL and lateral temporoparietal region, patients with lvPPA demonstrate asymmetric left greater than right hemisphere radiotracer retention, and patients with PCA are specifically targeted in the affected posterior brain regions (Fig. 1.10). Furthermore, the amount and area of tracer retention significantly correlate with the clinical severity of dementia and with a list of neuropsychological tests [149–151]. Interestingly, neocortical flortaucipir retention was found in some of the preclinical AD cases, but was rarely found in amyloid-negative cases [152, 153].

Tau imaging is not yet recommended for routine use in the clinical setting due to insufficient evidence.

1.2.3 Advanced MRI Techniques

1.2.3.1 Diffusion Tensor MRI
AD is associated with white matter abnormalities from early stages of the diseases [154]. A common finding in AD patients when compared with healthy controls is the alteration of both fractional anisotropy (FA) and mean diffusivity,

expression of axonal degeneration along white matter pathways due to the loss of cortical neurons. The mostly affected regions in AD are temporal lobes, posterior cingulum, and corpus callosum [155] with a typical posterior-to-anterior gradient in the severity of white matter abnormalities. Several studies showed that the pathological progression of the disease involved limbic, commissural, and associative tracts and suggested a progressive white matter degeneration within the AD continuum [156, 157], including amyloid-positive patients with subjective cognitive decline [158].

1.2.3.2 Functional MRI

Resting state functional MRI (RS fMRI) has the potential to detect subtle functional abnormalities in brain networks supporting complex cognitive processes that are progressively impaired over the course of AD [159]. RS fMRI in AD and MCI typically shows a dysfunction of the default mode network (DMN), which, in particular, consists of the posterior cingulate, inferior parietal, inferolateral temporal, anterior cingulate, prefrontal, and hippocampal regions [160]. In single-center studies, hypoconnectivity of the DMN had a good accuracy in differentiating AD patients from controls, with a sensitivity and specificity ranging from 70% to about 95% depending on the type of analysis [160]. The same marker demonstrated a high accuracy in distinguishing MCI converters to AD from stable MCI [161].

In the last decade, new advances in RS analysis techniques have shown the possibility of examining the overall structure of the brain network using graph analytical methods [159]. In particular, the functional connected brain network can be represented as a graph, consisting of nodes, and edges (or connections) between regions that are functionally linked. Specific parameters of the graph can be then assessed, such as clustering coefficient (expressing the level of connectedness of a graph), path length (indicating how efficiently information can be integrated between different systems), nodal strength (describing the number of connections of a node), and local efficiency (measuring the ability of a node to propagate information with the other nodes in a network). Different RS fMRI graph analysis studies have shown that the brain network is organized according to an efficient small-world organization. Small-world networks are known for their high level of local connectedness (i.e., high clustering coefficient), but still with a very short average travel distance (i.e., low path length) between the nodes of the network. As such, this organization combines a high-level local efficiency with a high level of global efficiency [159]. Several studies in AD and MCI patients revealed a decreased overall clustering and increased path length of the brain network in comparison to age-matched healthy controls, suggesting decreased efficiency of local information processing [162]. On the contrary, individuals with SCD may show a compensatory increase of nodal topological properties (e.g., nodal strength and clustering coefficient) mainly located in the DMN [163].

1.3 Clinical Case #1

A 53-years-old woman, known for hypothyroidism in replacement therapy, accessed the Memory Clinic complaining progressive short-term memory deficits in the last year. Differently from her previous habits, she has now to take note of her appointments and has some difficulties at focusing on her work, reason why her responsibilities have been recently rearranged.

The neurological examination resulted normal apart from difficulties at retaining new information. The neuropsychological assessment confirms deficits in short-term verbal and visuospatial memory, in association to modest impairment in visuospatial skills.

Routine hematology and serum biochemistry, comprehensive of thyroid function, vitamin B12, and folate dosage, were performed, showing normal results.

A visual inspection of coronal and axial T1-weighted MR sequences revealed a moderate atrophy of both hippocampi, as highlighted by a dilatation of temporal horns of lateral ventricles, and extending to the frontal and parietal lobes, bilaterally (Fig. 1.11a–c). FLAIR MR images showed only few white matter hyperintensities (Fig. 1.11d). Consistently, an FDG-PET evidenced a moderately reduced metabolism in MTL and lateral parietal and frontal lobes, bilaterally. Due to the young age, a lumbar puncture was also performed, showing no abnormalities regarding cell

Fig. 1.11 MRI scans from clinical case #1. (**a, b**) T1-weighted MR images showing bilateral hippocampal atrophy (circled). (**c**) T1-weighted MR scan showing lateral parietal and frontal atrophy (arrows). (**d**) FLAIR MR scan showing only modest signs of cerebrovascular disease

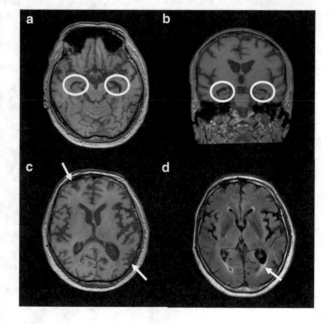

count, glucose and protein content. Conversely, dosage of CSF biomarkers demonstrated a typical AD profile (i.e., high tTau and pTau and low Aβ42).

A diagnosis of early-onset Alzheimer's disease dementia (high likelihood) with mild cognitive impairment was set according to NIA-AA Diagnostic Criteria [25].

1.4   Clinical Case #2

A 63-years-old man was accompanied by his wife at the Memory Clinic due to progressive difficulties in vision. He had been previously evaluated by an expert ophthalmologist, who did not found any eye alteration and addressed him to the neurologist.

The neurological examination outlined no motor or sensation abnormalities; modest bilateral ideomotor limb apraxia, some signs of optic ataxia, and environmental agnosia were identified. A complete neuropsychological evaluation revealed moderate visuospatial deficits, simultanagnosia, and modest oculomotor apraxia in addition to limb apraxia. The remaining cognitive domains appeared intact.

An MRI scan revealed bilateral (left > right) moderate atrophy of the occipital lobes, extending to parietal and temporal regions (Fig. 1.12). FDG-PET hypometabolism was consistently distributed.

A diagnosis of PCA was suspected, and a lumbar puncture was performed to ascertain subtended pathology. It showed a typical CSF AD profile (i.e., high tTau and pTau and low Aβ42), and a diagnosis of PCA-AD was set [20, 21].

Fig. 1.12 MRI scans from clinical case #2. (**a, b**) T1-weighted MR images showing moderate occipital and temporoparietal atrophy (left > right). (**c**) T1-weighted MR image showing enlargement of occipital sulci. (**d**) T2-weighted MR image showing moderate occipital and parietal atrophy and no white matter hyperintensities. *L* left, *R* right

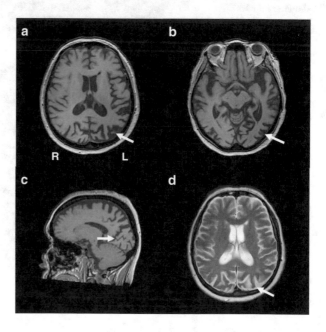

References

1. Qiu C, Kivipelto M, von Strauss E. Epidemiology of Alzheimer's disease: occurrence, determinants, and strategies toward intervention. Dialogues Clin Neurosci. 2009;11:111–28.
2. Crous-Bou M, Minguillon C, Gramunt N, Molinuevo JL. Alzheimer's disease prevention: from risk factors to early intervention. Alzheimers Res Ther. 2017;9:71.
3. International AsD. World Alzheimer report 2019: attitudes to dementia. London: Alzheimer's Disease International; 2019.
4. Takizawa C, Thompson PL, van Walsem A, Faure C, Maier WC. Epidemiological and economic burden of Alzheimer's disease: a systematic literature review of data across Europe and the United States of America. J Alzheimers Dis. 2015;43:1271–84.
5. Daviglus ML, Bell CC, Berrettini W, et al. National Institutes of Health state-of-the-science conference statement: preventing Alzheimer disease and cognitive decline. Ann Intern Med. 2010;153:176–81.
6. de Bruijn RF, Bos MJ, Portegies ML, et al. The potential for prevention of dementia across two decades: the prospective, population-based Rotterdam study. BMC Med. 2015;13:132.
7. Verghese PB, Castellano JM, Holtzman DM. Apolipoprotein E in Alzheimer's disease and other neurological disorders. Lancet Neurol. 2011;10:241–52.
8. Bateman RJ, Xiong C, Benzinger TL, et al. Clinical and biomarker changes in dominantly inherited Alzheimer's disease. N Engl J Med. 2012;367:795–804.
9. Braak H, Braak E. Staging of Alzheimer's disease-related neurofibrillary changes. Neurobiol Aging. 1995;16:271–8; discussion 278–84.
10. Braak H, Braak E. Neuropathological staging of Alzheimer-related changes. Acta Neuropathol. 1991;82:239–59.
11. Hardy J, Selkoe DJ. The amyloid hypothesis of Alzheimer's disease: progress and problems on the road to therapeutics. Science. 2002;297:353–6.
12. Schneider JA, Arvanitakis Z, Leurgans SE, Bennett DA. The neuropathology of probable Alzheimer disease and mild cognitive impairment. Ann Neurol. 2009;66:200–8.
13. Revesz T, McLaughlin JL, Rossor MN, Lantos PL. Pathology of familial Alzheimer's disease with Lewy bodies. J Neural Transm Suppl. 1997;51:121–35.
14. Nelson PT, Dickson DW, Trojanowski JQ, et al. Limbic-predominant age-related TDP-43 encephalopathy (LATE): consensus working group report. Brain. 2019;142:1503–27.
15. Winblad B, Palmer K, Kivipelto M, et al. Mild cognitive impairment—beyond controversies, towards a consensus: report of the International Working Group on Mild Cognitive Impairment. J Intern Med. 2004;256:240–6.
16. American Psychiatric Association. Diagnostic and statistical manual of mental disorders. Washington, DC: American Psychiatric Association; 2013.
17. Petersen RC, Lopez O, Armstrong MJ, et al. Practice guideline update summary: mild cognitive impairment: report of the guideline development, dissemination, and implementation subcommittee of the American Academy of neurology. Neurology. 2018;90:126–35.
18. Larrieu S, Letenneur L, Orgogozo JM, et al. Incidence and outcome of mild cognitive impairment in a population-based prospective cohort. Neurology. 2002;59:1594–9.
19. van Harten AC, Mielke MM, Swenson-Dravis DM, et al. Subjective cognitive decline and risk of MCI: the Mayo Clinic study of aging. Neurology. 2018;91:e300–12.
20. Crutch SJ, Lehmann M, Schott JM, et al. Posterior cortical atrophy. Lancet Neurol. 2012;11:170–8.
21. Crutch SJ, Schott JM, Rabinovici GD, et al. Consensus classification of posterior cortical atrophy. Alzheimers Dement. 2017;13:870–84.
22. Gorno-Tempini ML, Hillis AE, Weintraub S, et al. Classification of primary progressive aphasia and its variants. Neurology. 2011;76:1006–14.
23. Warren JD, Fletcher PD, Golden HL. The paradox of syndromic diversity in Alzheimer disease. Nat Rev Neurol. 2012;8:451–64.

24. Ossenkoppele R, Pijnenburg YA, Perry DC, et al. The behavioural/dysexecutive variant of Alzheimer's disease: clinical, neuroimaging and pathological features. Brain. 2015;138:2732–49.
25. Albert MS, DeKosky ST, Dickson D, et al. The diagnosis of mild cognitive impairment due to Alzheimer's disease: recommendations from the National Institute on Aging-Alzheimer's Association workgroups on diagnostic guidelines for Alzheimer's disease. Alzheimers Dement. 2011;7:270–9.
26. McKhann GM, Knopman DS, Chertkow H, et al. The diagnosis of dementia due to Alzheimer's disease: recommendations from the National Institute on Aging-Alzheimer's Association workgroups on diagnostic guidelines for Alzheimer's disease. Alzheimers Dement. 2011;7:263–9.
27. Dubois B, Feldman HH, Jacova C, et al. Research criteria for the diagnosis of Alzheimer's disease: revising the NINCDS-ADRDA criteria. Lancet Neurol. 2007;6:734–46.
28. Dubois B, Feldman HH, Jacova C, et al. Revising the definition of Alzheimer's disease: a new lexicon. Lancet Neurol. 2010;9:1118–27.
29. Knopman DS, DeKosky ST, Cummings JL, et al. Practice parameter: diagnosis of dementia (an evidence-based review)—report of the quality standards subcommittee of the American Academy of Neurology. Neurology. 2001;56:1143–53.
30. Jack CR Jr, Bennett DA, Blennow K, et al. A/T/N: an unbiased descriptive classification scheme for Alzheimer disease biomarkers. Neurology. 2016;87:539–47.
31. Jack CR Jr, Bennett DA, Blennow K, et al. NIA-AA research framework: toward a biological definition of Alzheimer's disease. Alzheimers Dement. 2018;14:535–62.
32. Chételat GA, Arbizu J, Barthel H, Garibotto V, Law I, Morbelli S, van de Giessen E, Agosta F. Amyloid-PET and ^{18}F-FDG-PET in the diagnostic investigation of Alzheimer's disease and other dementias. Lancet Neurol. 2020;19:951.
33. Thompson PM, Hayashi KM, de Zubicaray G, et al. Dynamics of gray matter loss in Alzheimer's disease. J Neurosci. 2003;23:994–1005.
34. Fox NC, Crum WR, Scahill RI, et al. Imaging of onset and progression of Alzheimer's disease with voxel-compression mapping of serial magnetic resonance images. Lancet. 2001;358:201–5.
35. Thompson PM, Mega MS, Woods RP, et al. Cortical change in Alzheimer's disease detected with a disease-specific population-based brain atlas. Cereb Cortex. 2001;11:1–16.
36. Teipel SJ, Bayer W, Alexander GE, et al. Progression of corpus callosum atrophy in Alzheimer disease. Arch Neurol. 2002;59:243–8.
37. Pasi M, Poggesi A, Pantoni L. The use of CT in dementia. Int Psychogeriatr. 2011;23(Suppl 2):S6–12.
38. Wattjes MP, Henneman WJ, van der Flier WM, et al. Diagnostic imaging of patients in a memory clinic: comparison of MR imaging and 64-detector row CT. Radiology. 2009;253:174–83.
39. Adduru V, Baum SA, Zhang C, et al. A method to estimate brain volume from head CT images and application to detect brain atrophy in Alzheimer disease. AJNR Am J Neuroradiol. 2020;41:224–30.
40. Braskie MN, Thompson PM. A focus on structural brain imaging in the Alzheimer's disease neuroimaging initiative. Biol Psychiatry. 2014;75:527–33.
41. Bush G, Luu P, Posner MI. Cognitive and emotional influences in anterior cingulate cortex. Trends Cogn Sci. 2000;4:215–22.
42. Dosenbach NU, Fair DA, Miezin FM, et al. Distinct brain networks for adaptive and stable task control in humans. Proc Natl Acad Sci U S A. 2007;104:11073–8.
43. Love S, Miners JS. Cerebrovascular disease in ageing and Alzheimer's disease. Acta Neuropathol. 2016;131:645–58.
44. Wardlaw JM, Brindle W, Casado AM, et al. A systematic review of the utility of 1.5 versus 3 Tesla magnetic resonance brain imaging in clinical practice and research. Eur Radiol. 2012;22:2295–303.

45. Gosche KM, Mortimer JA, Smith CD, Markesbery WR, Snowdon DA. Hippocampal volume as an index of Alzheimer neuropathology: findings from the Nun Study. Neurology. 2002;58:1476–82.

46. Csernansky JG, Hamstra J, Wang L, et al. Correlations between antemortem hippocampal volume and postmortem neuropathology in AD subjects. Alzheimer Dis Assoc Disord. 2004;18:190–5.

47. Frisoni GB, Fox NC, Jack CR Jr, Scheltens P, Thompson PM. The clinical use of structural MRI in Alzheimer disease. Nat Rev Neurol. 2010;6:67–77.

48. Scheltens P, Leys D, Barkhof F, et al. Atrophy of medial temporal lobes on MRI in "probable" Alzheimer's disease and normal ageing: diagnostic value and neuropsychological correlates. J Neurol Neurosurg Psychiatry. 1992;55:967–72.

49. Erkinjuntti T, Lee DH, Gao F, et al. Temporal lobe atrophy on magnetic resonance imaging in the diagnosis of early Alzheimer's disease. Arch Neurol. 1993;50:305–10.

50. Bresciani L, Rossi R, Testa C, et al. Visual assessment of medial temporal atrophy on MR films in Alzheimer's disease: comparison with volumetry. Aging Clin Exp Res. 2005;17:8–13.

51. Duara R, Loewenstein DA, Potter E, et al. Medial temporal lobe atrophy on MRI scans and the diagnosis of Alzheimer disease. Neurology. 2008;71:1986–92.

52. Diciotti S, Ginestroni A, Bessi V, et al. Identification of mild Alzheimer's disease through automated classification of structural MRI features. Annu Int Conf IEEE Eng Med Biol Soc. 2012;2012:428–31.

53. Frisoni GB, Jack CR. Harmonization of magnetic resonance-based manual hippocampal segmentation: a mandatory step for wide clinical use. Alzheimers Dement. 2011;7:171–4.

54. Frisoni GB, Jack CR Jr, Bocchetta M, et al. The EADC-ADNI harmonized protocol for manual hippocampal segmentation on magnetic resonance: evidence of validity. Alzheimers Dement. 2015;11:111–25.

55. Rowe CC, Ellis KA, Rimajova M, et al. Amyloid imaging results from the Australian Imaging, Biomarkers and Lifestyle (AIBL) study of aging. Neurobiol Aging. 2010;31:1275–83.

56. Apostolova LG, Morra JH, Green AE, et al. Automated 3D mapping of baseline and 12-month associations between three verbal memory measures and hippocampal atrophy in 490 ADNI subjects. NeuroImage. 2010;51:488–99.

57. Leow AD, Yanovsky I, Parikshak N, et al. Alzheimer's disease neuroimaging initiative: a one-year follow up study using tensor-based morphometry correlating degenerative rates, biomarkers and cognition. NeuroImage. 2009;45:645–55.

58. Carmichael O, Xie J, Fletcher E, et al. Localized hippocampus measures are associated with Alzheimer pathology and cognition independent of total hippocampal volume. Neurobiol Aging. 2012;33:1124, e1131–41.

59. Tosun D, Schuff N, Shaw LM, et al. Relationship between CSF biomarkers of Alzheimer's disease and rates of regional cortical thinning in ADNI data. J Alzheimers Dis. 2011;26(Suppl 3):77–90.

60. Stricker NH, Dodge HH, Dowling NM, et al. CSF biomarker associations with change in hippocampal volume and precuneus thickness: implications for the Alzheimer's pathological cascade. Brain Imaging Behav. 2012;6:599–609.

61. Scheltens P, Fox N, Barkhof F, De Carli C. Structural magnetic resonance imaging in the practical assessment of dementia: beyond exclusion. Lancet Neurol. 2002;1:13–21.

62. van der Flier WM, van Straaten EC, Barkhof F, et al. Medial temporal lobe atrophy and white matter hyperintensities are associated with mild cognitive deficits in non-disabled elderly people: the LADIS study. J Neurol Neurosurg Psychiatry. 2005;76:1497–500.

63. Shi F, Liu B, Zhou Y, Yu C, Jiang T. Hippocampal volume and asymmetry in mild cognitive impairment and Alzheimer's disease: meta-analyses of MRI studies. Hippocampus. 2009;19:1055–64.

64. Jack CR Jr, Petersen RC, Xu YC, et al. Prediction of AD with MRI-based hippocampal volume in mild cognitive impairment. Neurology. 1999;52:1397–403.

65. Apostolova LG, Dutton RA, Dinov ID, et al. Conversion of mild cognitive impairment to Alzheimer disease predicted by hippocampal atrophy maps. Arch Neurol. 2006;63:693–9.
66. Desikan RS, Cabral HJ, Fischl B, et al. Temporoparietal MR imaging measures of atrophy in subjects with mild cognitive impairment that predict subsequent diagnosis of Alzheimer disease. AJNR Am J Neuroradiol. 2009;30:532–8.
67. Yuan Y, Gu ZX, Wei WS. Fluorodeoxyglucose-positron-emission tomography, single-photon emission tomography, and structural MR imaging for prediction of rapid conversion to Alzheimer disease in patients with mild cognitive impairment: a meta-analysis. AJNR Am J Neuroradiol. 2009;30:404–10.
68. Stonnington CM, Chu C, Kloppel S, et al. Predicting clinical scores from magnetic resonance scans in Alzheimer's disease. NeuroImage. 2010;51:1405–13.
69. Dickerson BC, Wolk DA. Alzheimer's disease neuroimaging I. Dysexecutive versus amnesic phenotypes of very mild Alzheimer's disease are associated with distinct clinical, genetic and cortical thinning characteristics. J Neurol Neurosurg Psychiatry. 2011;82:45–51.
70. Evans MC, Barnes J, Nielsen C, et al. Volume changes in Alzheimer's disease and mild cognitive impairment: cognitive associations. Eur Radiol. 2010;20:674–82.
71. Bilgel M, An Y, Helphrey J, et al. Effects of amyloid pathology and neurodegeneration on cognitive change in cognitively normal adults. Brain. 2018;141:2475–85.
72. Chetelat G, Landeau B, Eustache F, et al. Using voxel-based morphometry to map the structural changes associated with rapid conversion in MCI: a longitudinal MRI study. NeuroImage. 2005;27:934–46.
73. Bozzali M, Filippi M, Magnani G, et al. The contribution of voxel-based morphometry in staging patients with mild cognitive impairment. Neurology. 2006;67:453–60.
74. Whitwell JL, Josephs KA, Murray ME, et al. MRI correlates of neurofibrillary tangle pathology at autopsy: a voxel-based morphometry study. Neurology. 2008;71:743–9.
75. Ferreira LK, Diniz BS, Forlenza OV, Busatto GF, Zanetti MV. Neurostructural predictors of Alzheimer's disease: a meta-analysis of VBM studies. Neurobiol Aging. 2011;32:1733–41.
76. Mitchell AJ, Beaumont H, Ferguson D, Yadegarfar M, Stubbs B. Risk of dementia and mild cognitive impairment in older people with subjective memory complaints: meta-analysis. Acta Psychiatr Scand. 2014;130:439–51.
77. Hafkemeijer A, Altmann-Schneider I, Oleksik AM, et al. Increased functional connectivity and brain atrophy in elderly with subjective memory complaints. Brain Connect. 2013;3:353–62.
78. Cherbuin N, Sargent-Cox K, Easteal S, Sachdev P, Anstey KJ. Hippocampal atrophy is associated with subjective memory decline: the PATH through life study. Am J Geriatr Psychiatry. 2015;23:446–55.
79. Striepens N, Scheef L, Wind A, et al. Volume loss of the medial temporal lobe structures in subjective memory impairment. Dement Geriatr Cogn Disord. 2010;29:75–81.
80. Frisoni GB, Pievani M, Testa C, et al. The topography of grey matter involvement in early and late onset Alzheimer's disease. Brain. 2007;130:720–30.
81. Canu E, Frisoni GB, Agosta F, et al. Early and late onset Alzheimer's disease patients have distinct patterns of white matter damage. Neurobiol Aging. 2012;33:1023–33.
82. van de Pol LA, Hensel A, Barkhof F, et al. Hippocampal atrophy in Alzheimer disease: age matters. Neurology. 2006;66:236–8.
83. Migliaccio R, Agosta F, Rascovsky K, et al. Clinical syndromes associated with posterior atrophy: early age at onset AD spectrum. Neurology. 2009;73:1571–8.
84. Whitwell JL, Jack CR Jr, Przybelski SA, et al. Temporoparietal atrophy: a marker of AD pathology independent of clinical diagnosis. Neurobiol Aging. 2011;32:1531–41.
85. Lehmann M, Rohrer JD, Clarkson MJ, et al. Reduced cortical thickness in the posterior cingulate gyrus is characteristic of both typical and atypical Alzheimer's disease. J Alzheimers Dis. 2010;20:587–98.
86. Whitwell JL, Przybelski SA, Weigand SD, et al. 3D maps from multiple MRI illustrate changing atrophy patterns as subjects progress from mild cognitive impairment to Alzheimer's disease. Brain. 2007;130:1777–86.

87. Bohnen NI, Djang DS, Herholz K, Anzai Y, Minoshima S. Effectiveness and safety of 18F-FDG PET in the evaluation of dementia: a review of the recent literature. J Nucl Med. 2012;53:59–71.

88. Herholz K, Schopphoff H, Schmidt M, et al. Direct comparison of spatially normalized PET and SPECT scans in Alzheimer's disease. J Nucl Med. 2002;43:21–6.

89. Perani D, Schillaci O, Padovani A, et al. A survey of FDG- and amyloid-PET imaging in dementia and GRADE analysis. Biomed Res Int. 2014;2014:785039.

90. Rice L, Bisdas S. The diagnostic value of FDG and amyloid PET in Alzheimer's disease—a systematic review. Eur J Radiol. 2017;94:16–24.

91. Bloudek LM, Spackman DE, Blankenburg M, Sullivan SD. Review and meta-analysis of biomarkers and diagnostic imaging in Alzheimer's disease. J Alzheimers Dis. 2011;26:627–45.

92. Spehl TS, Hellwig S, Amtage F, et al. Syndrome-specific patterns of regional cerebral glucose metabolism in posterior cortical atrophy in comparison to dementia with Lewy bodies and Alzheimer's disease—a [F-18]-FDG pet study. J Neuroimaging. 2015;25:281–8.

93. Nestor PJ, Altomare D, Festari C, et al. Clinical utility of FDG-PET for the differential diagnosis among the main forms of dementia. Eur J Nucl Med Mol Imaging. 2018;45:1509–25.

94. Nobili F, Arbizu J, Bouwman F, et al. European Association of Nuclear Medicine and European Academy of Neurology recommendations for the use of brain (18) F-fluorodeoxyglucose positron emission tomography in neurodegenerative cognitive impairment and dementia: Delphi consensus. Eur J Neurol. 2018;25:1201–17.

95. Mosconi L, Tsui WH, Herholz K, et al. Multicenter standardized 18F-FDG PET diagnosis of mild cognitive impairment, Alzheimer's disease, and other dementias. J Nucl Med. 2008;49:390–8.

96. Jagust W, Reed B, Mungas D, Ellis W, Decarli C. What does fluorodeoxyglucose PET imaging add to a clinical diagnosis of dementia? Neurology. 2007;69:871–7.

97. Mosconi L, Andrews RD, Matthews DC. Comparing brain amyloid deposition, glucose metabolism, and atrophy in mild cognitive impairment with and without a family history of dementia. J Alzheimers Dis. 2013;35:509–24.

98. Murayama N, Iseki E, Fujishiro H, et al. Detection of early amnestic mild cognitive impairment without significantly objective memory impairment: a case-controlled study. Psychogeriatrics. 2010;10:62–8.

99. Arbizu J, Festari C, Altomare D, et al. Clinical utility of FDG-PET for the clinical diagnosis in MCI. Eur J Nucl Med Mol Imaging. 2018;45:1497–508.

100. Anchisi D, Borroni B, Franceschi M, et al. Heterogeneity of brain glucose metabolism in mild cognitive impairment and clinical progression to Alzheimer disease. Arch Neurol. 2005;62:1728–33.

101. Santangelo R, Masserini F, Agosta F, et al. CSF p-tau/Abeta42 ratio and brain FDG-PET may reliably detect MCI "imminent" converters to AD. Eur J Nucl Med Mol Imaging. 2020;47:3152.

102. Drzezga A, Lautenschlager N, Siebner H, et al. Cerebral metabolic changes accompanying conversion of mild cognitive impairment into Alzheimer's disease: a PET follow-up study. Eur J Nucl Med Mol Imaging. 2003;30:1104–13.

103. Mosconi L, Perani D, Sorbi S, et al. MCI conversion to dementia and the APOE genotype: a prediction study with FDG-PET. Neurology. 2004;63:2332–40.

104. Knopman DS, Jack CR Jr, Wiste HJ, et al. Selective worsening of brain injury biomarker abnormalities in cognitively normal elderly persons with beta-amyloidosis. JAMA Neurol. 2013;70:1030–8.

105. Knopman DS, Jack CR Jr, Lundt ES, et al. Role of beta-amyloidosis and neurodegeneration in subsequent imaging changes in mild cognitive impairment. JAMA Neurol. 2015;72:1475–83.

106. Kemp PM, Holmes C, Hoffmann SM, et al. Alzheimer's disease: differences in technetium-99m HMPAO SPECT scan findings between early onset and late onset dementia. J Neurol Neurosurg Psychiatry. 2003;74:715–9.

107. Rabinovici GD, Furst AJ, Alkalay A, et al. Increased metabolic vulnerability in early-onset Alzheimer's disease is not related to amyloid burden. Brain. 2010;133:512–28.

108. Laforce R Jr, Tosun D, Ghosh P, et al. Parallel ICA of FDG-PET and PiB-PET in three conditions with underlying Alzheimer's pathology. Neuroimage Clin. 2014;4:508–16.
109. Madhavan A, Whitwell JL, Weigand SD, et al. FDG PET and MRI in logopenic primary progressive aphasia versus dementia of the Alzheimer's type. PLoS One. 2013;8:e62471.
110. Nestor PJ, Caine D, Fryer TD, Clarke J, Hodges JR. The topography of metabolic deficits in posterior cortical atrophy (the visual variant of Alzheimer's disease) with FDG-PET. J Neurol Neurosurg Psychiatry. 2003;74:1521–9.
111. Kas A, de Souza LC, Samri D, et al. Neural correlates of cognitive impairment in posterior cortical atrophy. Brain. 2011;134:1464–78.
112. Woodward MC, Rowe CC, Jones G, Villemagne VL, Varos TA. Differentiating the frontal presentation of Alzheimer's disease with FDG-PET. J Alzheimers Dis. 2015;44:233–42.
113. Laforce R Jr, Buteau JP, Paquet N, et al. The value of PET in mild cognitive impairment, typical and atypical/unclear dementias: a retrospective memory clinic study. Am J Alzheimers Dis Other Dement. 2010;25:324–32.
114. Herholz K, Ebmeier K. Clinical amyloid imaging in Alzheimer's disease. Lancet Neurol. 2011;10:667–70.
115. Wong DF, Rosenberg PB, Zhou Y, et al. In vivo imaging of amyloid deposition in Alzheimer disease using the radioligand 18F-AV-45 (florbetapir [corrected] F 18). J Nucl Med. 2010;51:913–20.
116. Rinne JO, Wong DF, Wolk DA, et al. [(18)F]Flutemetamol PET imaging and cortical biopsy histopathology for fibrillar amyloid beta detection in living subjects with normal pressure hydrocephalus: pooled analysis of four studies. Acta Neuropathol. 2012;124:833–45.
117. Rowe CC, Ackerman U, Browne W, et al. Imaging of amyloid beta in Alzheimer's disease with 18F-BAY94-9172, a novel PET tracer: proof of mechanism. Lancet Neurol. 2008;7:129–35.
118. Johnson KA, Minoshima S, Bohnen NI, et al. Update on appropriate use criteria for amyloid PET imaging: dementia experts, mild cognitive impairment, and education. J Nucl Med. 2013;54:1011–3.
119. Clark CM, Schneider JA, Bedell BJ, et al. Use of florbetapir-PET for imaging beta-amyloid pathology. JAMA. 2011;305:275–83.
120. Clark CM, Pontecorvo MJ, Beach TG, et al. Cerebral PET with florbetapir compared with neuropathology at autopsy for detection of neuritic amyloid-beta plaques: a prospective cohort study. Lancet Neurol. 2012;11:669–78.
121. Braskie MN, Klunder AD, Hayashi KM, et al. Plaque and tangle imaging and cognition in normal aging and Alzheimer's disease. Neurobiol Aging. 2010;31:1669–78.
122. Ossenkoppele R, Zwan MD, Tolboom N, et al. Amyloid burden and metabolic function in early-onset Alzheimer's disease: parietal lobe involvement. Brain. 2012;135:2115–25.
123. Cho H, Seo SW, Kim JH, et al. Amyloid deposition in early onset versus late onset Alzheimer's disease. J Alzheimers Dis. 2013;35:813–21.
124. Lee JH, Kim SH, Kim GH, et al. Identification of pure subcortical vascular dementia using 11C-Pittsburgh compound B. Neurology. 2011;77:18–25.
125. Leyton CE, Villemagne VL, Savage S, et al. Subtypes of progressive aphasia: application of the International Consensus Criteria and validation using beta-amyloid imaging. Brain. 2011;134:3030–43.
126. Rabinovici GD, Rosen HJ, Alkalay A, et al. Amyloid vs FDG-PET in the differential diagnosis of AD and FTLD. Neurology. 2011;77:2034–42.
127. Rabinovici GD, Furst AJ, O'Neil JP, et al. 11C-PIB PET imaging in Alzheimer disease and frontotemporal lobar degeneration. Neurology. 2007;68:1205–12.
128. Forsberg A, Engler H, Almkvist O, et al. PET imaging of amyloid deposition in patients with mild cognitive impairment. Neurobiol Aging. 2008;29:1456–65.
129. Lim YY, Maruff P, Pietrzak RH, et al. Effect of amyloid on memory and non-memory decline from preclinical to clinical Alzheimer's disease. Brain. 2014;137:221–31.
130. Okello A, Koivunen J, Edison P, et al. Conversion of amyloid positive and negative MCI to AD over 3 years: an 11C-PIB PET study. Neurology. 2009;73:754–60.

131. Grundman M, Pontecorvo MJ, Salloway SP, et al. Potential impact of amyloid imaging on diagnosis and intended management in patients with progressive cognitive decline. Alzheimer Dis Assoc Disord. 2013;27:4–15.
132. Marcus C, Mena E, Subramaniam RM. Brain PET in the diagnosis of Alzheimer's disease. Clin Nucl Med. 2014;39:e413–22; quiz e423–6
133. Iaccarino L, Sala A, Perani D. Alzheimer's disease neuroimaging I. Predicting long-term clinical stability in amyloid-positive subjects by FDG-PET. Ann Clin Transl Neurol. 2019;6:1113–20.
134. Ostrowitzki S, Deptula D, Thurfjell L, et al. Mechanism of amyloid removal in patients with Alzheimer disease treated with gantenerumab. Arch Neurol. 2012;69:198–207.
135. Morris JC, Price JL. Pathologic correlates of nondemented aging, mild cognitive impairment, and early-stage Alzheimer's disease. J Mol Neurosci. 2001;17:101–18.
136. Ng S, Villemagne VL, Berlangieri S, et al. Visual assessment versus quantitative assessment of 11C-PIB PET and 18F-FDG PET for detection of Alzheimer's disease. J Nucl Med. 2007;48:547–52.
137. Formaglio M, Costes N, Seguin J, et al. In vivo demonstration of amyloid burden in posterior cortical atrophy: a case series with PET and CSF findings. J Neurol. 2011;258:1841–51.
138. Kambe T, Motoi Y, Ishii K, Hattori N. Posterior cortical atrophy with [11C] Pittsburgh compound B accumulation in the primary visual cortex. J Neurol. 2010;257:469–71.
139. Tenovuo O, Kemppainen N, Aalto S, Nagren K, Rinne JO. Posterior cortical atrophy: a rare form of dementia with in vivo evidence of amyloid-beta accumulation. J Alzheimers Dis. 2008;15:351–5.
140. Rosenbloom MH, Alkalay A, Agarwal N, et al. Distinct clinical and metabolic deficits in PCA and AD are not related to amyloid distribution. Neurology. 2011;76:1789–96.
141. Rabinovici GD, Jagust WJ, Furst AJ, et al. Abeta amyloid and glucose metabolism in three variants of primary progressive aphasia. Ann Neurol. 2008;64:388–401.
142. de Souza LC, Corlier F, Habert MO, et al. Similar amyloid-beta burden in posterior cortical atrophy and Alzheimer's disease. Brain. 2011;134:2036–43.
143. Xia CF, Arteaga J, Chen G, et al. [(18)F]T807, a novel tau positron emission tomography imaging agent for Alzheimer's disease. Alzheimers Dement. 2013;9:666–76.
144. Chien DT, Bahri S, Szardenings AK, et al. Early clinical PET imaging results with the novel PHF-tau radioligand [F-18]-T807. J Alzheimers Dis. 2013;34:457–68.
145. Chien DT, Szardenings AK, Bahri S, et al. Early clinical PET imaging results with the novel PHF-tau radioligand [F18]-T808. J Alzheimers Dis. 2014;38:171–84.
146. Marquie M, Siao Tick Chong M, Anton-Fernandez A, et al. [F-18]-AV-1451 binding correlates with postmortem neurofibrillary tangle Braak staging. Acta Neuropathol. 2017;134:619–28.
147. Vogel JW, Mattsson N, Iturria-Medina Y, et al. Data-driven approaches for tau-PET imaging biomarkers in Alzheimer's disease. Hum Brain Mapp. 2019;40:638–51.
148. Schwarz AJ, Yu P, Miller BB, et al. Regional profiles of the candidate tau PET ligand 18F-AV-1451 recapitulate key features of Braak histopathological stages. Brain. 2016;139:1539–50.
149. Mattsson N, Insel PS, Donohue M, et al. Predicting diagnosis and cognition with (18) F-AV-1451 tau PET and structural MRI in Alzheimer's disease. Alzheimers Dement. 2019;15:570–80.
150. Ossenkoppele R, Schonhaut DR, Scholl M, et al. Tau PET patterns mirror clinical and neuroanatomical variability in Alzheimer's disease. Brain. 2016;139:1551–67.
151. Okamura N, Harada R, Ishiki A, et al. The development and validation of tau PET tracers: current status and future directions. Clin Transl Imaging. 2018;6:305–16.
152. Sperling R, Mormino E, Johnson K. The evolution of preclinical Alzheimer's disease: implications for prevention trials. Neuron. 2014;84:608–22.
153. Pontecorvo MJ, Devous MD Sr, Navitsky M, et al. Relationships between flortaucipir PET tau binding and amyloid burden, clinical diagnosis, age and cognition. Brain. 2017;140:748–63.

154. Kavcic V, Ni H, Zhu T, Zhong J, Duffy CJ. White matter integrity linked to functional impairments in aging and early Alzheimer's disease. Alzheimers Dement. 2008;4:381–9.
155. Sexton CE, Kalu UG, Filippini N, Mackay CE, Ebmeier KP. A meta-analysis of diffusion tensor imaging in mild cognitive impairment and Alzheimer's disease. Neurobiol Aging. 2011;32:2322.e5–18.
156. Pievani M, Agosta F, Pagani E, et al. Assessment of white matter tract damage in mild cognitive impairment and Alzheimer's disease. Hum Brain Mapp. 2010;31:1862–75.
157. Zhang X, Sun Y, Li W, et al. Characterization of white matter changes along fibers by automated fiber quantification in the early stages of Alzheimer's disease. Neuroimage Clin. 2019;22:101723.
158. Teipel SJ, Kuper-Smith JO, Bartels C, et al. Multicenter tract-based analysis of microstructural lesions within the Alzheimer's disease spectrum: association with amyloid pathology and diagnostic usefulness. J Alzheimers Dis. 2019;72:455–65.
159. Verstraete E, van den Heuvel MP, Veldink JH, et al. Motor network degeneration in amyotrophic lateral sclerosis: a structural and functional connectivity study. PLoS One. 2010;5:e13664.
160. Agosta F, Pievani M, Geroldi C, et al. Resting state fMRI in Alzheimer's disease: beyond the default mode network. Neurobiol Aging. 2012;33:1564–78.
161. Petrella JR, Sheldon FC, Prince SE, Calhoun VD, Doraiswamy PM. Default mode network connectivity in stable vs progressive mild cognitive impairment. Neurology. 2011;76:511–7.
162. Supekar K, Menon V, Rubin D, Musen M, Greicius MD. Network analysis of intrinsic functional brain connectivity in Alzheimer's disease. PLoS Comput Biol. 2008;4:e1000100.
163. Chen H, Sheng X, Luo C, et al. The compensatory phenomenon of the functional connectome related to pathological biomarkers in individuals with subjective cognitive decline. Transl Neurodegener. 2020;9:21.

Vascular Cognitive Impairment

2

Contents

2.1 Clinicopathological Findings

The term vascular cognitive impairment (VCI) refers to a syndrome that includes any cognitive disorder in which the blood flow impairment due to a cerebrovascular disease has a key role in the definition of the clinical picture. The degree of cognitive impairment may be variable, ranging from subjective cognitive decline (SCD)

© Springer Nature Switzerland AG 2021
M. Filippi, F. Agosta, *Imaging Dementia*,
https://doi.org/10.1007/978-3-030-66773-3_2

to dementia, including mild cognitive impairment (MCI) [1]. This kind of cognitive impairment is usually defined by two clinical scenarios [2]:

1. cognitive impairment that follows a clinically diagnosed stroke;
2. progressive cognitive decline without a clear clinical history of stroke.

2.1.1   Epidemiology

VCI is a very common form of cognitive impairment; it is the second most common form of dementia, which only follows Alzheimer's disease (AD) in terms of incidence and prevalence [3]. Even though VCI is a common disorder, the diagnosis of pure vascular dementia is uncommon. Vascular pathology alone causes less than 10% of dementia cases, while it is an important contributive factor in multiple-etiology (also termed "mixed") dementia, mainly associated to AD pathology, accounting for approximately 30–40% of all dementia cases [4].

2.1.2   Etiology and Pathophysiology

VCI is caused by diseases of the cerebral vascular system. The common feature of these diseases is the alteration of the normal function of brain vessels, leading to brain ischemia or loss of vascular wall integrity causing hemorrhage [5]. According to the underlying pathophysiology, VCI can be considered as secondary to:

- Large vessels disease (LVD) or post-stroke dementia: ischemic stroke of any cause (i.e., large artery atherosclerosis or cardioembolism) may lead to VCI. This may be caused by a single strategically placed infarct, for instance medial frontal lobe or medial temporal lobe strokes, or by multiple infarcts producing a cumulative brain damage [6].
- Small vessel disease (SVD): it is the most common neuropathologic correlate in both pure vascular and mixed dementia [7]. The main types of SVD are arteriolosclerosis and cerebral amyloid angiopathy (CAA) [8]. Arteriolosclerosis is the most common form, characterized by alterations in the walls of small arteries and loss of vascular integrity [8], mainly located in subcortical brain regions, such as the basal ganglia and corona radiata. CAA is the second most common type of cerebral SVD, caused by the deposition of amyloid-β in small arteries of leptomeninges and cerebral cortex, which leads to the loss of vascular integrity mostly restricted to the cortical brain regions [9].
- Others: rare causes of VCI include genetic disorders, such as cerebral autosomal dominant arteriopathy with subcortical infarcts and leukoencephalopathy (CADASIL) [10], Fabry's disease [11], and vasculitides [12, 13].

2.1.3 Risk Factors

The risk factors related to cardiovascular and cerebrovascular diseases are also related to VCI. In population-based studies, the major risk factors for VCI are age, hypertension, diabetes, elevated total cholesterol levels, smoking, coronary artery disease, and atrial fibrillation [14–18]. As protective factor, the cognitive reserve is still an under-recognized factor, even though occupational attainment and higher education are associated with lower risk of developing cognitive impairment in vascular pathology [19].

2.1.4 Clinical Picture

The degree of cognitive impairment in VCI is highly variable, according to the underlying etiology. The cognitive profile of post-stroke dementia includes the prominent impairment of executive functions, with relative sparing of episodic memory [20]. This cognitive clinical picture is enriched by other cortical signs caused by the stroke event, including aphasia and apraxia. Stroke location and severity account for the wide variation in cognitive profiles that is typically observed across subjects. In some cases, cognitive impairment may be mostly evident in the stroke acute phase and then improve during the stroke recovery process, although a systematic review showed that about 10% of patients will develop dementia after stroke in a 1–4-year time range [21]. Regarding patients with VCI without a clinically evident stroke event, the cognitive profile is usually characterized by impairment in executive functions and processing speed [22], often associated with a less prominent deficit in memory and other functions [23]. CAA usually presents a similar impairment of attention and executive functions, with associated episodic memory deficits, even though to a lesser degree than what is typically observed in AD cases [24]. In most cases of VCI, the progression of cognitive impairment assumes the pattern of a series of stepwise declines, but, in some cases, it may worsen slowly and constantly [25], mimicking the course of a neurodegenerative disease. Cognitive disorders due to vascular pathology are frequently accompanied by motor and neuropsychiatric signs. The motor impairment is characterized mainly of slowing and gait impairment and may lead to a syndrome described as lower body parkinsonism [26]. The neuropsychiatric picture is defined by depression, abulia, apathy, psychosis with delusions or hallucinations [27].

Some clinical features may indicate a specific underlying etiology. For example, CADASIL is characterized by a typical syndrome including transient ischemic attacks, recurrent strokes, ataxia, cognitive decline and dementia, in patients who frequently present a history of migraine, usually with aura [28]. Fabry's disease is also characterized by subtle cognitive impairment associated with transient ischemic attacks and strokes, occurring in patients with a history of cardiac disease (left ventricular hypertrophy, rhythm abnormalities, and small coronary vessel disease), renal insufficiency and progressive length-dependent small fiber neuropathy with acroparesthesia, and loss of cold and warm perception [12]. The clinical picture of central nervous system vasculitides is widely variable, with cognitive dysfunction often associated with a history of subacute or chronic headache and aseptic meningitis [13, 29]. In these cases, cerebral ischemic episodes involve different vascular beds, and there is evidence of inflammatory changes in the cerebrospinal fluid (CSF) if lumbar puncture is performed [29].

2.1.5   Diagnostic Criteria

Diagnostic criteria for VCI have been defined by several organizations, including the American Heart Association/American Stroke Association criteria (AHA/ASA) [30], the Diagnostic and Statistical Manual of Mental Disorders-V criteria (DSM-V) [31], and the International Society of Vascular Behavioral and Cognitive Disorders (VAS-COG) [6]. Conceptually, these criteria share a similar basis:

- The presence of cerebrovascular disease must be sustained by a clinical history of stroke and/or its demonstration on neuroimaging evaluations;
- Cerebrovascular disease must be sufficiently severe to explain the degree of cognitive impairment;
- VCI is classified in different degrees of severity corresponding, with different terminology, to MCI and dementia, and the diagnosis does not require the presence of memory deficits;
- Neuroimaging has a key role in the definition of probable VCI: in all three sets of criteria, even when the clinical criteria are met, the absence of a neuroimaging study showing sufficiently severe vascular disease allows only a diagnosis of possible VCI.

Table 2.1 summarizes and compares the three sets of diagnostic criteria.

2.2   Neuroimaging

2.2.1   Conventional Neuroimaging Techniques

According to the diagnostic criteria of VCI, it is clear that neuroimaging is a fundamental method for the in vivo assessment of brain vascular damage, providing important information regarding diagnosis and prognosis of this condition. As already mentioned in the previous paragraphs, during the diagnostic workup of patients with suspected VCI, the overlap with neurodegenerative pathology must be considered. In fact, the presence of cerebral vascular damage has been demonstrated as an independent risk factor for the development of dementia and greater

Table 2.1 Key aspects of diagnostic criteria for VCI

AHA/ASA [30]	VAS-COG society [6]	DSM-V [31]
Cognitive criteria		
Discriminates between vascular mild cognitive impairment and dementia	Discriminates between mild and major vascular cognitive disorder	Discriminates between mild and major vascular neurocognitive disorder
Criteria for probable vascular cognitive impairment		

Imaging evidence of cerebrovascular disease and either:
• Clear temporal relationship between vascular event (i.e., clinically evident stroke) and onset of cognitive deficits OR
• Clear relationship in the severity and pattern of cognitive impairment and the presence of diffuse, subcortical cerebrovascular disease pathology
 	
No clinical history suggesting a non-vascular cognitive disorder
	Either:
	• Cognitive deficit onset after one or more strokes or physical signs consistent with stroke OR
	• Evidence of cognitive decline in speed information processing, complex attention, frontal executive functions, accompanied by one or more: gait disturbances, urinary symptoms, personality or mood changes.
	
	Neuroimaging evidence of either large vessel infarct, strategically placed single infarct(s) or intracerebral hemorrhage(s), multiple (almost two) lacunar infarcts outside the brainstem or extensive confluent white matter lesions.
	Absence of evidence of non-vascular cognitive, medical, psychiatric or neurologic disorder sufficient to explain impairment
		The criteria for mild or major neurocognitive disorders are met.
		Probable vascular neurocognitive disorder is diagnosed if one of the following is present; otherwise possible vascular neurocognitive disorder should be diagnosed:
		• Clinical criteria are supported by neuroimaging evidence of significant parenchymal injury attributed to cerebrovascular disease (neuroimaging supported).
		  OR
		• The neurocognitive syndrome is temporally related to one or more documented cerebrovascular events.
		  OR
		• Both clinical and genetic (e.g., cerebral autosomal dominant arteriopathy with subcortical infarcts and leukoencephalopathy) evidence of cerebrovascular disease is present.

Criteria for possible vascular cognitive impairment		
Meets criteria in absence of temporal relationship, insufficient information (i.e., no neuroimaging studies available), severe aphasia preclude cognitive assessment, evidence of neurodegenerative condition	Meets criteria except that neuroimaging is not available	Clinical criteria are met, but neuroimaging is not available and the temporal relationship is not established
Classification when other potential causes are present (i.e., mixed disease)		
There is evidence of other neurodegenerative condition	The criteria for probable or possible Alzheimer's disease are met	

Abbreviations: *AHA/ASA* American Heart Association/American Stroke Association, *DSM-V* Diagnostic and Statistical Manual of Mental Disorders-5 criteria, *VAS-COG* The International Society of Vascular Behavioural and Cognitive Disorders

impairment in most cognitive domains in cases with concomitant AD pathology [32]. Therefore, brain atrophy patterns consistent with concomitant neurodegenerative causes of dementia (see dedicated chapters in the present book) should also be assessed when VCI is suspected.

The main structural neuroimaging techniques used in the clinical setting are computed tomography (CT) and magnetic resonance imaging (MRI). Whenever possible, MRI is preferred to CT for both routine clinical use and research purposes, due to the higher sensitivity and specificity to detect pathological imaging correlates [33].

2.2.1.1 Computed Tomography

CT remains an important technique in the emergency setting and is mainly performed to exclude the presence of hemorrhages, brain tumors, or other stroke mimics. CT can also show the presence of indirect sign of ischemic stroke or the presence of pre-existent vascular lesions. The main features of cerebral vascular pathology that can be visualized by CT are focal ischemic or hemorrhagic lesions, as well as extensive alterations of the white matter. If CT is used to study VCI, the investigator should obtain a thin-section volume sequence of 5 mm or less, without contrast, covering the whole brain [34]. In addition, reconstruction of images in all the three planes is recommended, in particular the coronal plane reconstruction, for the optimal visualization of the hippocampus [34].

2.2.1.2 Magnetic Resonance Imaging

MRI is the first-choice neuroimaging technique that allows the identification of brain alterations related to vascular pathology with a higher level of detail compared to CT (see Table 2.2 for a comparison between the two techniques in this context). MRI is preferred over CT unless there are absolute contraindications to MRI, such as the presence of a cardiac not MRI-conditional pacemaker. The minimum MRI protocol should include [34] the following:

- DWI sequence to detect acute ischemic lesions for up to several weeks after a cerebrovascular event with highest sensitivity;
- T2-weighted images and fluid-attenuated inversion recovery (FLAIR) images to detect white matter alterations, such as white matter hyperintensities of presumed vascular origin and lacunar lesions; because of the advantage derived from using FLAIR sequences, which suppress CSF signal, the use of T2-FLAIR sequences facilitates the discrimination of enlarged perivascular spaces or lacunes from white matter hyperintensities, even though FLAIR sequences have a low sensitivity for lesions in the infratentorial regions [35];
- T1-weighted images with thin slices and multiplanar reconstruction to assess the severity of infracts and to detect regional atrophy, e.g., coronal T1-weighted images parallel to the long axis of the hippocampus;
- T2*-weighted gradient recall-echo (GRE) or susceptibility-weighted imaging (SWI) to detect the signal derived from microbleeds and superficial siderosis.

Table 2.2 Comparison between MRI and CT capability of brain vascular damage identification

Lesion	Detectable by CT?	MRI sequences used for detection	Superiority of each method
Large infarcts	Yes	T2	MRI = CT
Small and lacunar infarcts	Yes	T1, T2 and/or FLAIR	MRI > CT
White matter lesions	Yes	FLAIR	MRI > CT
Microbleeds	No	SWI	MRI only
Enlarged perivascular spaces	Yes	T2	MRI > CT
Global atrophy	Yes	T1 and/or FLAIR	MRI = CT
Structural integrity of the white matter	No	DTI	MRI only; should be considered in research setting only
Cortical microinfarcts	No	DWI	3T MRI only; should be considered in research setting only

Reprinted by permission from Springer Nature: Macmillan Publishers Limited, Nature Reviews Disease Primers, Vascular cognitive impairment, van der Flier WM, Skoog I, Schneider JA, Pantoni L, Mok V, Chen CLH, Scheltens P. © 2018
MRI > CT denotes MRI is superior to CT; MRI = CT denotes MRI and CT have similar performance
Abbreviations: *DTI* diffusion tensor imaging, *DWI* diffusion-weighted imaging, *FLAIR* fluid-attenuated inversion recovery, *SWI* susceptibility-weighted imaging, *T1* T1-weighted images, *T2* T2-weighted images

Regarding the field strength, the use of a 3T (Tesla) scanner might be preferred, but images of a modern 1.5T MR scanner also have an acceptable definition and due to the wider availability represent a good choice for clinical use [36].

2.2.2 Structural Imaging Correlates of VCI

Even though the pathological basis of VCI may be schematically divided into LVD and SVD, in the clinical practice these two entities are often coexistent, and the subsequent neuroimaging picture is composed of a complex patchwork of radiological signs. The main feature of LVD is the presence of large ischemic lesions, identified by CT or MRI, which may be expression of a previous clinically evident stroke or silent brain infarction. The vascular contribution to cognitive impairment and dementia due to SVD has several imaging biomarkers that can be best evaluated on MRI studies, such as prominent perivascular spaces and cerebral microbleeds, and others visible also on CT scans, although with a lower definition, such as white matter damage and lacunes.

The radiologic definitions of brain changes caused by brain vascular disease are provided by the Standards for Reporting Vascular Changes on Neuroimaging (STRIVE) criteria [34]. The most important signs are described in the following paragraphs and summarized in Fig. 2.1.

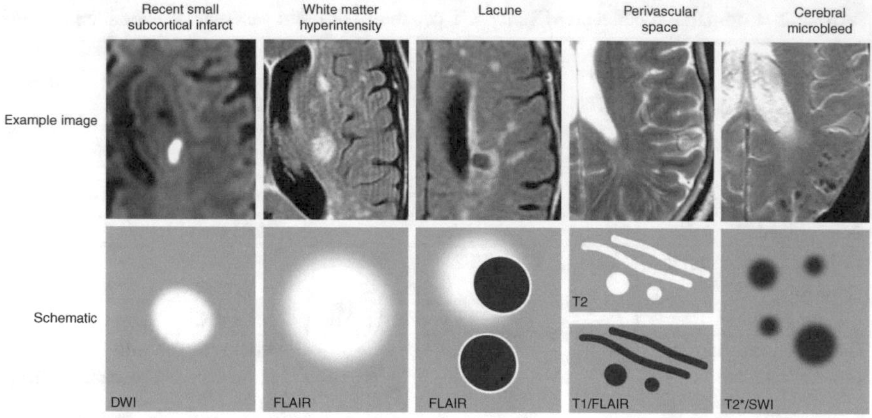

	Recent small subcortical infarct	White matter hyperintensity	Lacune	Perivascular space	Cerebral microbleed
Example image					
Schematic	DWI	FLAIR	FLAIR	T1/FLAIR (T2)	T2*/SWI
Usual diameter	≤20 mm	Variable	3–15 mm	≤2 mm	≤10 mm
Comment	Best identified on DWI	Located in white matter	Usually have hyperintense rim	Most linear without hyperintense rim	Detected on GRE seq., round or ovoid, blooming
DWI	↑	↔	↔(↓)	↔	↔
FLAIR	↑	↑	↓	↓	↔
T2	↑	↑	↑	↑	↔
T1	↓	↔(↓)	↓	↓	↔
T2*-weighted GRE	↔	↑	↔ (↓ if haemorrhage)	↔	↓↓

↑ Increased signal ↓ Decreased signal ↔ ISO-intense signal

Fig. 2.1 MRI appearance of cerebral vascular lesions associated with cognitive impairment, according to the Standards for Reporting Vascular Changes on Neuroimaging (STRIVE) classification criteria. (Reprinted from The Lancet Neurology, 12, Wardlaw JM, Smith EE, Biessels GJ, et al., Neuroimaging standards for research into small vessel disease and its contribution to ageing and neurodegeneration, 822–838. © (2013), with permission from Elsevier)

2.2.2.1 Large Vessel Disease (Large Ischemic Lesions)

The impact of stroke on cognition depends on lesion location [37] and even a single infarct may have a key role in cognitive decline, affecting global cognition or specific cognitive domains, including language, memory, executive, attentive, and visuospatial functions. The presence of an acute ischemic lesion may be visualized on MR studies as a hyperintensity on FLAIR and DWI with a correspondent hypointensity on the apparent diffusion coefficient (ADC) map (Fig. 2.2) [38]. In early stages, CT only allows the identification of indirect stroke signs, as a hypodensity of the damaged brain tissue becomes apparent 6–24 h after the clinical onset [39]. Whereas T2/FLAIR hyperintensity of ischemic lesions is generally persistent, DWI and ADC signal progressively change over time, so that chronic lesions (i.e., >3 weeks from appearance) are eventually isointense on DWI and hyperintense on ADC map [38]. T1-weighted hypointensity also characterizes subacute and chronic cerebral infarcts, although cortical necrosis may cause transient hyperintensity in subacute phases (1–3 weeks after clinical onset) [38].

Cognitive impairment is often recognized in the weeks and months following an ischemic event [40], as an ischemic stroke can be associated with either an acute

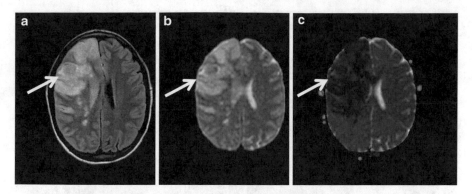

Fig. 2.2 MRI appearance of an acute large cerebral infarct. FLAIR scan (**a**, arrow) shows hyperintensity in the middle cerebral artery field. Diffusion-weighted study shows restriction of water molecules, with a resulting hyperintensity on DWI map (**b**) and hypointensity on ADC map (**c**) in the corresponding regions

change in cognition or a slower cognitive decline over time [40]. As recommended by international guidelines, cognitive assessment should be part of the routine follow-up after an acute ischemic event in clinical practice [41]. In the clinical practice, a change in cognition due to LVD may also become apparent in the absence of a clinically evident stroke. In this setting, the main etiology is tied to the presence of a silent brain infarction identified by an *ex post* neuroimaging assessment. The overall prevalence of silent brain infarctions increases with age and appears to range between 8% and 28% in the general population [42]. Although silent brain infarctions are common findings in elderly patients [43], these are not currently considered as benign in nature, as they are often associated with a severe evolution of cognitive dysfunction and psychiatric disorders, as well as higher risk of subsequent cerebrovascular events [44, 45]. Radiologically, silent brain infarctions are characterized by a hypodensity with negative mass effect on CT scans and low T1-weighted signal and high T2-weighted signal on MRI scans [38]; these alterations are mostly chronic, and are therefore usually associated with high ADC values and variable DWI signal, which progressively decrease over time [38].

The degree of VCI derived from a single stroke event is strictly related to the location of the infarction. Many studies identified the basal ganglia, internal capsule, thalamus, corpus callosum, angular gyrus, cingulate cortex, and frontal subcortical regions as strategic regions for post-stroke cognitive impairment, mainly if the lesions are located in the dominant hemisphere [46].

2.2.2.2 Small Vessel Disease

White Matter Hyperintensities of Presumed Vascular Origin
White matter alterations are a common finding in VCI, detectable both with CT and MRI studies (Fig. 2.3). The first historical observation of white matter lesions was made with CT scans, identified as a hypodense confluent alteration of white matter

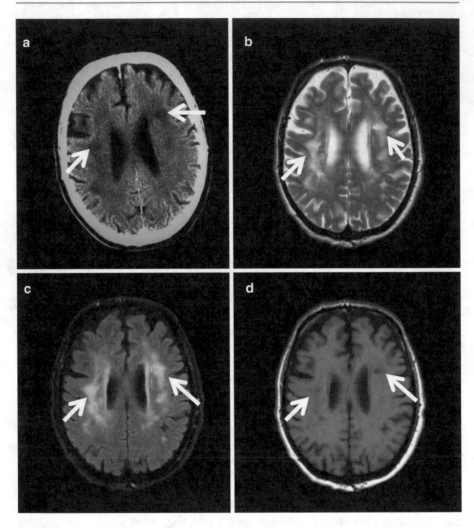

Fig. 2.3 White matter alterations of presumed vascular origin. (**a**) CT scan shows confluent hypodensities in the periventricular and deep white matter (arrows). White matter hyperintensities on the T2-weighted and FLAIR scans (**b** and **c**, arrows) correspond to hypointense signal alterations on T1-weighted image (**d**, arrows)

and named "leukoaraiosis" [47]. Later, with the widespread use of MRI, this kind of alterations were better characterized and identified as white matter hyperintensities (WMHs), due to their hyperintense appearance on T2-weighted images [34]. WMHs are a common finding in non-demented adults aged over 65 years, with a prevalence up to 90%, with various degree of severity [48]. The association between increasing age and WMHs has been well defined [49–51]. The term "of presumed vascular origin" was added to distinguish this kind of lesions from the white matter damage associated with other causes (e.g., inflammatory diseases) [34].

WMHs are the most common abnormalities seen on MRI scans, identified as diffuse and hyperintense lesions on T2-weighted images, mainly in the periventricular regions and in the centrum semiovale (Fig. 2.3b) [52]. Because of the hyperintensity of the CSF in T2-weighted images, FLAIR images may be used to null the fluid signal, which is useful to identify correctly WMHs in regions adjacent to the liquoral spaces (Fig. 2.3c). On T1-weighted images, a signal alteration may be seen in correspondent areas: if these areas are isointense on T1-weighted imaging, they represent an area of incomplete infarction; if these areas show an hypointensity, they are caused by a complete infarction with tissue destruction (Fig. 2.3d) [53].

According to their location, WMHs are further divided into periventricular, i.e., located next to the lateral ventricles, and deep (or subcortical), i.e., distinct and separate from the ventricles [54, 55]. Pathological studies suggested that WMHs are characterized by gliosis and discontinuous ependyma, with demyelination and axonal damage [56]. An histopathologic-radiologic correlation study demonstrated that FLAIR and T2-weighted images may lead to overestimate the pathologic demyelination in the periventricular regions and underestimate the demyelination in deep regions [57]. Many studies tried to better characterize these lesions, suggesting the higher clinical relevance of WMHs located in the deep white matter in the definition of cognitive impairment and mood alteration [58, 59]. In some cases, characteristic localizations of WMHs may indicate specific causes of VCI. For instance, the main characteristic feature of CADASIL on MRI is the presence of large and confluent WMHs affecting the subcortical U fibers, with a typical involvement of the external capsules and temporal poles (Fig. 2.4) [54, 60].

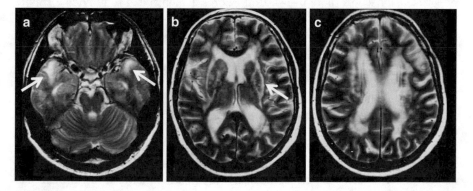

Fig. 2.4 Main characteristic features of cerebral autosomal dominant arteriopathy with subcortical infarcts and leukoencephalopathy (CADASIL) on T2-weighted MRI scans of two patients: (**a**) typical involvement of the temporal poles (arrows); and (**b, c**) large and confluent WMHs affecting the subcortical U fibers, with a typical involvement of the external capsules (arrow). (Reproduced from Yousry TA, Seelos K, Mayer M, et al. Characteristic MR lesion pattern and correlation of T1 and T2 lesion volume with neurologic and neuropsychological findings in cerebral autosomal dominant arteriopathy with subcortical infarcts and leukoencephalopathy (CADASIL). AJNR Am J Neuroradiol 1999; 20:91–100, with permission)

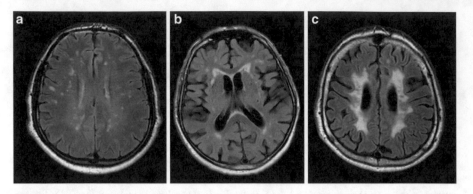

Fig. 2.5 Fazekas scale of white matter hyperintensities (WMHs) on FLAIR MRI. (**a**) Grade 1: multiple punctate WMHs. (**b**) Grade 2: bridging of punctate WMHs leading to confluent lesions. (**c**) Grade 3: widespread confluent WMH

For the clinical practice, many studies provided simple rating scales to easily classify the severity of white matter damage using FLAIR and T2-weighted MR sequences. The most used are the Fazekas score [55] and the more elaborated Scheltens score [61]. The Fazekas scale is more easily applicable and grades the severity of WMHs from 0 to 3—grade 0 representing occasional or non-punctate WMH; grade 1, multiple punctate WMHs (Fig. 2.5); grade 2, bridging of punctate WMHs leading to confluent lesions; and grade 3, widespread confluent WMH— whereas the Scheltens scale sums 4 subscores in a semiquantitative way—periventricular (0–6), deep white matter (0–24), basal ganglia, and infratentorial hyperintensity scores (both 0–24). Both scores demonstrated to provide a simple visual rating score to evaluate the global load of WMHs, which correlates with global functional decline in elderly subjects [62] and the risk of developing dementia [22]. A large European study that involved people aged over 65 years without disability showed that the presence of severe confluent white matter lesions at baseline was associated with a high rate of progression to disability over a 3-year period [63]. Regarding the relationship with cognition, higher WMH load has been related to worse cognitive performance, both general [64, 65] and domain-specific, especially in executive functions [66], processing speed [67], and episodic memory [68]. In longitudinal studies, non-demented subjects showed that greater WMH load correlated with a faster cognitive decline over time [65]. Similarly, a more severe WMH burden has been associated with greater functional impairment due to cognitive and balance disturbances in cognitively impaired subjects with mild parkinsonian signs [69, 70].

Due to the high prevalence of WMHs among both cognitively impaired and cognitively normal subjects, it is difficult to establish a clear threshold for the definition of "abnormal" vascular WMHs for a given age that might be directly related to an evident clinical picture. Although some early studies suggested a threshold of 10 cm^2 [71] or 25% of total white matter [72] as surely pathological, to date, no clear evidence is available for such definition.

Lacunes

Lacunes are complete and focal infarcts that measure less than 2 cm in diameter, caused by the atherosclerotic obliteration of deep small vessels [73]. They are the second most common neuroradiological correlate of brain vascular pathology seen in VCI cases. Similar to WMHs, lacunes are associated with increasing age. Data from a large population study showed that the incidence of silent infarctions in a population of healthy subjects aged more than 65 was of 26% and 83% of these were classified as lacunar infarctions [74]. For the detection of small lacunes, MRI is more sensitive than CT (Fig. 2.6) [53]. Lacunar infarcts on CT scans appear as a small ovoid hypodensity usually located in the deep white matter (Fig. 2.6a). On MRI scans, they appear as a defined round or ovoid cavity, filled with fluid and hyperintense in T2-weighted images, measuring usually between 3 and 15 mm in

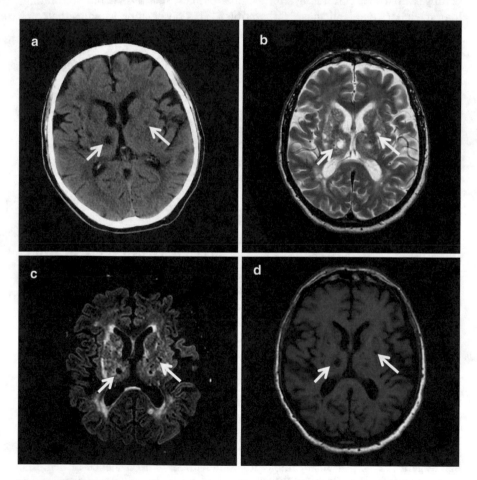

Fig. 2.6 Multiple lacunes of vascular origin occurring in the basal ganglia region and thalami (indicated by arrows). (**a**) CT scan, (**b**) T2-weighted MR image, (**c**) FLAIR MR image, and (**d**) T1-weighted MR image

diameter (Fig. 2.6b) [34]. On FLAIR sequences, a hyperintense peripheral rim can often be observed, surrounding a hypointense core, although the identification of this rim is non-specific, as it can be observed also in periventricular spaces (Fig. 2.6c) [34]. On T1-weighted images, lacunes appear as hypointense lesions (Fig. 2.6d). The distinction between perivascular spaces and lacunes is an important issue in neuroradiology: most studies use the minimal cut-off of 3 mm to differentiate lacunes from perivascular spaces and the upper limit of 15 mm to distinguish lacunes from larger ischemic lesions [75].

Lacunes and WMHs are often observed together in the setting of a VCI, due to the common pathogenetic origin (i.e., SVD) and the shared risk factors. Pathologically, lacunes are the result of lypohyalinosis and microatheroma of penetrating arteries, due to systemic hypertension and diabetes [76]. These changes are mainly seen in deep perforating arteries and arterioles, such as thalamo-perforating, long medullary and lenticulostriate arterioles. This observation explains the common localization of lacunes in the basal ganglia, upper two-thirds of the putamen, internal capsule, and thalamus [53]. The identification of sharply defined lacunar infarcts in the periventricular and subcortical white matter, external capsule, thalamus, and basal ganglia may be indicative of CADASIL [77].

Lacunar infarcts have been associated with poor cognitive performance and cognitive impairment. Some studies showed that multiple lacunar strokes in deep regions are associated with executive and attentive dysfunctions [67, 78]. Regarding other domain-specific deficits, silent lacunar infarcts located in the thalamus were related to decline in memory performance, while non-thalamic lacunes were related to impairment in psychomotor speed [79]. Overall, lacunes appear to be an important neuropathological contributor to VCI.

Perivascular Spaces

Perivascular spaces, also called Virchow-Robin spaces, are subpial interstitial spaces surrounding the penetrating arteries and arterioles [80]. When small, they may be not visible on conventional MRI, but with high-field scanner (i.e., 3 T or higher) they appear more evident [81]. Perivascular spaces are filled with fluid that follows the course of a vessel through the gray or white matter. They appear as a small, oval hyperintensity with a well-defined smooth margin, isointense to CSF, in most cases not larger than 3 mm, commonly seen along the path of the lenticulostriate arteries entering the basal ganglia or along the perforating medullary arteries entering the cortical gray matter (Fig. 2.7). These spaces show no contrast enhancement and are usually bilateral [53]. In the basal ganglia, these spaces may be particularly prominent, with a diameter up to 20 mm [34]. This observation explains why they can be confused for lacunar infarcts.

Dilated perivascular spaces are thought to be caused by increased vascular permeability with subsequent fluid exudation and obstruction of the lymphatic drainage system [82, 83]. In histopathologic studies, there is no evidence of necrosis, immune cells, or tissue debris [53]. They appear to be associated with similar risk factors as for other correlates of cerebrovascular disease, mainly with systemic hypertension [84]. In studies that considered perivascular spaces, a major issue is

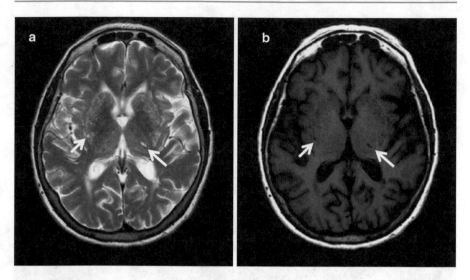

Fig. 2.7 MRI appearance of enlarged perivascular spaces (indicated by arrows), mainly located in the basal ganglia, on a (**a**) T2-weighted scan and (**b**) T1-weighted scan

represented by the differences between MRI scanners, as the identification of these spaces heavily depends on MRI resolution and strength of the field used [81]. Due to this issue, data on perivascular spaces in large population-based studies is limited, and the reported prevalence varies significantly in the literature. However, the load of perivascular spaces is significantly associated with increasing age [85]. They appear to be a frequent sign in neuroradiological exams also in the healthy population, as about 80% of healthy subject showed mild, 11% moderate, and 3% severe visualization of perivascular spaces in the basal ganglia on MRI scans [86].

Not only the epidemiological data appear to be limited but also the association between cognition and perivascular spaces has yet to be exhaustively explored. Some studies suggest that healthy elderly male individuals with dilated perivascular spaces appear to have worse cognitive function [87] and faster cognitive decline, mainly in processing speed [88]. The presence of multiple enlarged perivascular spaces in the basal ganglia is called "état criblé," which has been related to the development of cognitive decline and movement disorders, mainly mild parkinsonian syndromes [89].

Cerebral Microbleeds

Cerebral microbleeds (CMBs) are defined as small, rounded, hypointense foci not attributable to vessels, calcifications, or other pathologic conditions, visible on T2*-weighted GRE or SWI images (Fig. 2.8). They are related to the presence of a bleeding-prone microangiopathy leading to the deposition of hemosiderin. The development of MRI techniques with the capability to detect magnetic susceptibility allowed the recognition of this kind of lesions [90]. Sequences such as GRE or SWI are characterized by an intense signal loss in region containing paramagnetic

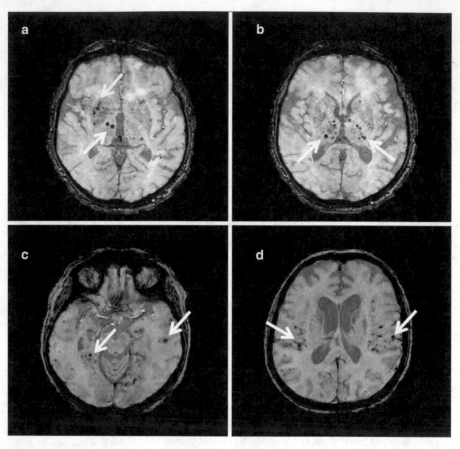

Fig. 2.8 SWI MR scans show the presence of multiple cerebral microbleeds (indicated by arrows) related to different etiologies. Deep location, such as in the thalamus or basal ganglia, is suggestive for hypertensive vasculopathy (**a, b**). Lobar location is typical of cerebral amyloid angiopathy (**c, d**)

elements, such as products derived from blood degradation: deoxyhemoglobin, metahemoglobin, and hemosiderin. After the extravasation of red blood cells, hemoglobin undergoes a degradation process in the perivascular space and parenchyma [75]. Histopathologically, a CMB is a focal accumulation of macrophages that contains hemosiderin [91]. Different etiologies are related to different CMB localizations: a deep location, such as in the thalamus or basal ganglia, is suggestive for hypertensive vasculopathy (Fig. 2.8a, b), whereas a cortical (also named "lobar") location is typical of CAA (Fig. 2.8c, d) [90]. The presence of multiple, diffuse microhemorrhagic foci on GRE and SWI sequences is indicative of CADASIL as etiology of VCI [77].

According to several epidemiological studies, increasing age is related to higher odd of having CMBs, with a prevalence ranging from 4.7% to 24.4% [92–94]. This wide range derives from demographic heterogeneity between cohorts and differences in MRI protocols. In fact, it has been shown that the introduction of SWI has improved the quantification of CMBs, when compared with conventional GRE imaging [95]. Higher magnetic fields are also associated with enhanced CMB detection [96, 97]. CMBs are a common finding in aging patients without a known neurologic disease, even though patients with CAA have a higher prevalence of CMBs [98–100]. Apart from age, the major risk factors are systemic hypertension (mainly for deep microbleeds) and male sex [99–101]. The presence of an Apolipoprotein ε4 allele also increases the risk of developing lobar CMBs, particularly in the parietal cortical regions [102].

Regarding the relationship between CMBs and cognitive functioning, there are two main hypotheses. According to some, CMBs might interfere with the normal wiring of connections between different brain regions which have a role in cognition [103]. However, it has also been suggested that CMBs might represent an epiphenomenon of more widespread brain vascular pathology without a real pathophysiological role per se as CMBs are rarely observed as isolated lesions [104]. In fact, although the presence of one or more CMBs has been associated with poorer cognitive performance regardless the age, current evidence is relatively limited, particularly in non-demented subjects [92, 104]. To date, there is no clear correspondence between the detection of CMBs on MRI and cognitive decline in healthy control subjects [98], and the correlation between the location of CMBs and cognitive symptoms is controversial [105].

Brain Atrophy

Brain atrophy occurs in many disorders, including VCI, and may be widespread or focal (i.e., only in some regions such as the hippocampus), symmetrical or asymmetrical. Brain atrophy is a common and paraphysiological age-related finding, with a great variability between subjects, represented by cortical thinning and diminished brain volume with enlargement of the ventricles and subarachnoid spaces, quantifiable on both CT and MRI scans (Fig. 2.9). In the context of VCI, the neuropathologic substrate of atrophy includes neuronal loss secondary to ischemic damage and subsequent cortical thinning [106]. Many imaging studies showed a relationship between the presence and severity of brain vascular disease and brain atrophy, particularly, of the corpus callosum, basal ganglia, midbrain, and hippocampus, in addition to focal cortical thinning in brain regions connected to subcortical infarcts [107, 108]. However, in the context of VCI, the evaluation of patterns of brain atrophy is mostly useful to identify overlapping neurodegenerative causes of cognitive dysfunction.

2.2.3 Molecular Imaging

As highlighted in the previous paragraphs, conventional MRI is the first choice for the identification of neuroimaging markers of VCI. However, functional molecular imaging techniques may provide some additional clues for a diagnostic definition of this condition.

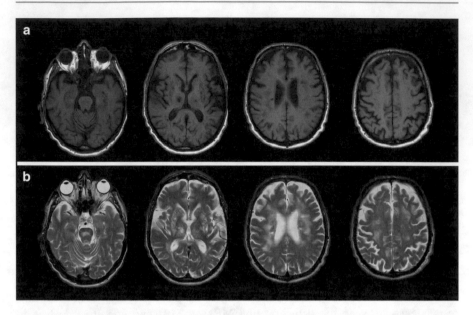

Fig. 2.9 T1-weighted (**a**) and T2-weighted (**b**) MR scans show the presence of widespread brain atrophy, with cortical thinning and enlargement of the ventricles and subarachnoid spaces in a patient with vascular cognitive impairment

For the diagnostic workup of VCI and other cognitive disorders, FDG-PET can support differential diagnosis by visualizing metabolic alterations in typically affected brain regions. PET studies in patients with probable AD typically show hypometabolism in the temporal, parietal, and frontal association regions, with relative sparing of sensorimotor cortex, basal ganglia, and cerebellum (see Chap. 1 and Fig. 1.5) [109]. By contrast, in VCI patients a different pattern is usually reported, with a significant reduction of metabolism in several cortical regions, mainly middle frontal cortex, temporoparietal cortex, cerebellum, basal ganglia, and brainstem, with a distinctive involvement of subcortical structures and primary sensorimotor cortex (Fig. 2.10) [110]. The use of a metabolic ratio (metabolism in association areas divided by that of areas mainly affected in VCI) was found to be lower in AD compared to VCI patients, with a parallel decline of this metabolic ratio with increasing severity of cognitive impairment [110]. However, the total volume of regions which showed hypometabolism did not differ significantly between AD and VCI, and it was not possible to define a single region able to differentiate the two conditions [110].

Additional PET tracers permit the study of selective receptor system damage. Amyloid tracers including ^{11}C-labeled Pittsburgh Compound B (PiB), ^{18}F-florbetaben, and ^{18}F-florbetapir can detect brain amyloid-β deposition, therefore indicating in vivo VCI subjects with concomitant AD pathology [111]. In fact, recent studies

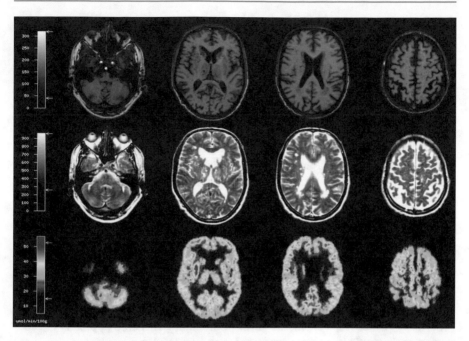

Fig. 2.10 T1-weighted and T2-weighted MR and FDG-PET images in vascular cognitive impairment associated with multiple small infarcts, lacunes, and widespread white matter hyperintensities. FDG-PET images show diffuse impairment of metabolism in both hemispheres, in the basal ganglia, thalamus, and cerebellum. (Reprinted from J Neurol Sci, 322, Heiss WD, Zimmermann-Meinzingen S, PET imaging in the differential diagnosis of vascular dementia, 268–273, © (2012), with permission from Elsevier)

using amyloid PET demonstrated that approximately 30% of VCI individuals have significant concurrent AD pathology [112, 113], which has been associated with more rapid cognitive decline [29]. This is important in order to identify those subjects with VCI that would benefit from AD-targeted therapies. Amyloid PET has been also used as a promising marker of a CAA etiology in cases of intracerebral hemorrhages [109].

Another interesting PET tracer for the study of VCI is ^{11}C[R]-PK11195, developed to measure the activity of microglia as marker of neuroinflammation [114]. Ischemia-induced neuroinflammation can trigger a neurodegenerative process of fiber tracts, even in tracts not directly affected by ischemia, compromising large-scale brain networks [115]. In the context of post-stroke dementia, the activation of microglia in the affected hemisphere was found to highly correlate with cognitive performance [116]. However, further studies are needed to support a clinical relevance of PET markers of neuroinflammation for VCI patients.

2.2.4   Advanced MRI Techniques

2.2.4.1 Diffusion Tensor MRI

In cognitively normal subjects, greater WMH load has been associated with loss of microstructural white matter integrity shown by diffusion tensor (DT) MRI also outside the borders of visible lesions, suggesting an involvement of normal-appearing white matter driven by vascular pathology, which correlates with the severity of subthreshold cognitive alterations [117, 118]. DT MRI alterations in VCI extending beyond visible lesions are likely due to increased extracellular fluid, as a result of increased permeability of the blood–brain barrier secondary to small vessel injury [119]. Consistently, in SVD patients, measures of cognitive impairment were significantly correlated with alterations of DT MRI measures (i.e., fractional anisotropy and diffusivity metrics) in white matter tracts of cerebral hemispheres, including the corpus callosum, intra-thalamic white matter tracts, and superior cerebellar peduncle [120, 121], indicating DT MRI as an independent, sensitive marker of VCI.

Structural connectivity studies based on DT MRI showed that network efficiency is lower in patients with vascular pathology compared to control subjects and that these advanced metrics are closely correlated to the degree of cognitive impairment [122, 123]. Moreover, a decreased network efficiency was able to predict the conversion to dementia in patients diagnosed with VCI [124].

In the future, these metrics may serve as additional biomarkers for early SVD and related cognitive impairment.

2.2.4.2 Functional MRI

Given that pathological damage to subcortical structures is a key element of VCI, functional MRI (fMRI) is an ideal technique in order to explore the impact of functional disconnection between brain regions on cognition. In fact, this approach has been shown to discriminate VCI cases from control subjects, demonstrating functional alterations that were associated with cognitive test scores [125–127]. Significant associations between local WMH load and changes in brain functional connectivity which, in turn, are related to cognitive deficits of SVD patients suggest a primary role of cerebrovascular pathology in disrupting functional networks in these patients [128, 129], particularly when compared with MCI due to underlying AD pathology [128]. Although further studies are warranted, fMRI represents a promising approach to explore subtle rearrangements due to vascular pathology in patients with cognitive impairment.

2.3   Clinical Case #1

A 71-year-old man, with personal history of active smoking and hypertension, presented with significant mental slowness, apathy, attention, and concentration difficulties. The first cognitive symptoms (i.e., an isolated impairment of recent memory) had appeared at the age of 68 and subsequently progressed over the following years.

In addition, he developed gait difficulties, characterized by small steps and slow walking.

The neurological examination revealed a mild and symmetric parkinsonism, mainly affecting the inferior limbs, in the absence of resting tremor. Deep tendon reflexes were enhanced in lower limbs and bilateral pyramidal signs with extensor plantar reflexes were present. At the neuropsychological evaluation, cognition was severely affected, with a marked impairment in short-term memory and attention. The Mini Mental Status Examination (MMSE) was 16/30, and he was totally dependent in the activities of daily living.

Routine hematology and serum biochemistry, including coagulation testing, thyroid function and levels of vitamin B12, and folate were performed, showing normal results.

MRI scan revealed an extensive pattern of confluent white matter hyperintensities on FLAIR images in the periventricular regions bilaterally, associated with lacunes in basal ganglia and thalami (Fig. 2.11a). Some degree of cortical atrophy was also observed, especially in frontal and temporal lobes, involving also the hippocampus (Fig. 2.11b). A lumbar puncture was performed, showing no abnormalities regarding cell count, glucose, and protein levels. Cerebrospinal fluid (CSF) examination showed a typical AD protein profile: high total-tau and phospho-tau, low amyloid-β.

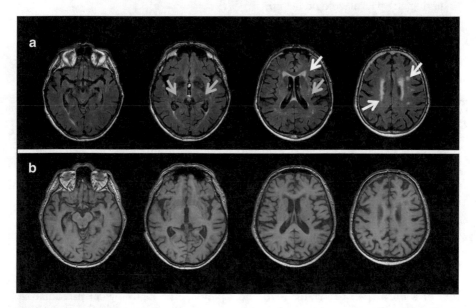

Fig. 2.11 Case #1: Series of FLAIR MR scans (**a**) that show confluent white matter hyperintensities in periventricular and deep regions (white arrows), associated with enlarged perivascular spaces (orange arrows) and lacunes (green arrow) in the basal ganglia regions. Correspondent T1-weighted MR images (**b**) are shown to highlight the presence of cortical thinning, mainly located in frontal and temporoparietal lobes (including the hippocampi, white arrows), with an overall decrease in brain volume and a wider representation of sulci in these areas

According to VCI diagnostic criteria [6, 30, 31], the patient fulfilled a diagnosis of probable vascular dementia. In consideration of the clinical onset, the MRI picture reporting hippocampal atrophy, and the CSF biomarkers that confirmed the presence of AD pathology, the patient's clinical picture represents a typical case of mixed dementia, in which a primitive neurodegenerative disorder is associated with cognitive decline due to cerebral vascular disease. Mixed vascular and AD dementia represents the second most common form of dementia in terms of incidence and prevalence [3], and is therefore an important condition to be considered for the differential diagnostic process.

2.4   Clinical Case #2

A 48-years-old man showed a 2-year history of gradually progressive memory loss and a 1-year history of diminished attention and social activity, depression, and loss of interest in life and his hobbies. His wife reported that, in the last 6 months, he misidentified his relatives and could not remember the names of other people. The clinical picture worsened over the last 2 years. The patient's medical history included hypertension. He was also an ex-smoker. His family history was positive for cerebral ischemic infarction (father) and cognitive decline of unknown etiology (mother). The patient has a sister suffering from migraine. The patient was not assuming any pharmacologic therapy.

At physical examination, the patient's blood pressure was 160/100 mmHg, 75 bpm. His orientation, memory, comprehension, and calculation were impaired. The cranial nerve examination showed no abnormalities. Deep tendon reflexes were normal, not associated with any pyramidal sign. The sensory examination was normal. During the visit, the patient scored 18/30 at MMSE and 10/30 on the Montreal Cognitive Assessment (MoCA). Laboratory assessment of blood, thyroid, liver and kidney functions, vitamin B12, and folate showed no abnormalities.

Brain MRI showed multiple punctate WMHs in the periventricular white matter, bilateral basal ganglia, thalamus, external capsule, centrum semiovale, and bilateral frontoparietal subcortical regions (Fig. 2.12a–f). These signal abnormalities were hyperintense on T2-weighted images and markedly hypointense on T1-weighted images. The scan showed also a ventricular enlargement and atrophy, mainly located in the frontal lobes. In the periventricular and deep regions, two lacunes were also identifiable (Fig. 2.12d).

According to the described findings, the patient was diagnosed with VCI due to small vessel disease.

In the following year, the cognitive decline progressed. The patient's wife led him to a third level center for a second opinion. The neurological examination showed no differences compared to the previous one, but the patient scored 15/30 on MMSE and 8/30 on MoCA. The MRI scan was repeated, showing an increased extension of the previously identified signal alterations involving also the temporal poles. An FDG-PET was also performed and showed decreased tracer uptake in the

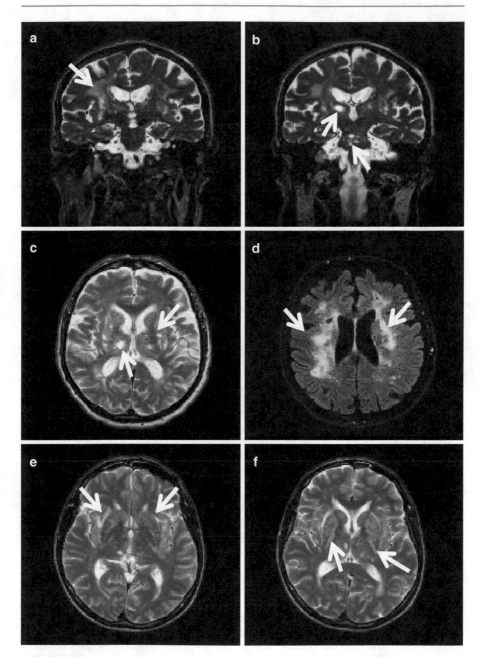

Fig. 2.12 Case #2: Coronal (**a**, **b**) and axial (**c**) T2-weighted MR images showing widespread confluent white matter hyperintensities with focus on pons (**b**), basal ganglia and thalami (**a–c**), and associated evidence of multiple lacunar infarcts (**c**). Axial FLAIR MR scan shows the involvement of centrum semiovale (**d**). Axial T2-weighted images showing confluent hyperintensities involving both external (**e**, **f**) and internal capsule (**f**). Alterations are indicated by arrows

left frontal and temporal lobes, thalamus, and basal ganglia. Subsequently, analysis of the *NOTCH3* gene on chromosome 19 was performed, showing a substitution in exon 33 involving cysteine, leading to the diagnosis of cerebral autosomal dominant arteriopathy with subcortical infarcts and leukoencephalopathy (CADASIL).

References

1. van der Flier WM, Skoog I, Schneider JA, et al. Vascular cognitive impairment. Nat Rev Dis Primers. 2018;4:18003.
2. Smith EE. Clinical presentations and epidemiology of vascular dementia. Clin Sci (Lond). 2017;131:1059–68.
3. Neuropathology Group of the Medical Research Council Cognitive Function and Ageing Study (MRC CFAS). Pathological correlates of late-onset dementia in a multicentre, community-based population in England and Wales. Lancet. 2001;357:169–75.
4. Schneider JA, Arvanitakis Z, Bang W, Bennett DA. Mixed brain pathologies account for most dementia cases in community-dwelling older persons. Neurology. 2007;69:2197–204.
5. Iadecola C. The pathobiology of vascular dementia. Neuron. 2013;80:844–66.
6. Sachdev P, Kalaria R, O'Brien J, et al. Diagnostic criteria for vascular cognitive disorders: a VASCOG statement. Alzheimer Dis Assoc Disord. 2014;28:206–18.
7. Kalaria RN. Neuropathological diagnosis of vascular cognitive impairment and vascular dementia with implications for Alzheimer's disease. Acta Neuropathol. 2016;131:659–85.
8. Pantoni L. Cerebral small vessel disease: from pathogenesis and clinical characteristics to therapeutic challenges. Lancet Neurol. 2010;9:689–701.
9. Vinters HV, Gilbert JJ. Cerebral amyloid angiopathy: incidence and complications in the aging brain. II. The distribution of amyloid vascular changes. Stroke. 1983;14:924–8.
10. Dichgans M, Mayer M, Uttner I, et al. The phenotypic spectrum of CADASIL: clinical findings in 102 cases. Ann Neurol. 1998;44:731–9.
11. Loeb J, Feldt-Rasmussen U, Madsen CV, Vogel A. Cognitive impairments and subjective cognitive complaints in Fabry disease: a Nationwide study and review of the literature. JIMD Rep. 2018;41:73–80.
12. Kozora E, Arciniegas DB, Filley CM, et al. Cognitive and neurologic status in patients with systemic lupus erythematosus without major neuropsychiatric syndromes. Arthritis Rheum. 2008;59:1639–46.
13. Hajj-Ali RA, Saygin D, Ray E, et al. Long-term outcomes of patients with primary angiitis of the central nervous system. Clin Exp Rheumatol. 2019;37(Suppl 117):45–51.
14. Sharp SI, Aarsland D, Day S, Sonnesyn H, Ballard C. Hypertension is a potential risk factor for vascular dementia: systematic review. Int J Geriatr Psychiatry. 2011;26:661–9.
15. Hebert R, Lindsay J, Verreault R, et al. Vascular dementia: incidence and risk factors in the Canadian study of health and aging. Stroke. 2000;31:1487–93.
16. Hassing LB, Johansson B, Nilsson SE, et al. Diabetes mellitus is a risk factor for vascular dementia, but not for Alzheimer's disease: a population-based study of the oldest old. Int Psychogeriatr. 2002;14:239–48.
17. Reitz C, Tang MX, Luchsinger J, Mayeux R. Relation of plasma lipids to Alzheimer disease and vascular dementia. Arch Neurol. 2004;61:705–14.
18. Lackland DT, Roccella EJ, Deutsch AF, et al. Factors influencing the decline in stroke mortality: a statement from the American Heart Association/American Stroke Association. Stroke. 2014;45:315–53.
19. Murray AD, Staff RT, McNeil CJ, et al. The balance between cognitive reserve and brain imaging biomarkers of cerebrovascular and Alzheimer's diseases. Brain. 2011;134:3687–96.
20. Sachdev PS, Brodaty H, Valenzuela MJ, et al. The neuropsychological profile of vascular cognitive impairment in stroke and TIA patients. Neurology. 2004;62:912–9.

21. Pendlebury ST, Rothwell PM. Prevalence, incidence, and factors associated with pre-stroke and post-stroke dementia: a systematic review and meta-analysis. Lancet Neurol. 2009;8:1006–18.
22. Debette S, Markus HS. The clinical importance of white matter hyperintensities on brain magnetic resonance imaging: systematic review and meta-analysis. BMJ. 2010;341:c3666.
23. de Groot JC, de Leeuw FE, Oudkerk M, et al. Cerebral white matter lesions and cognitive function: the Rotterdam Scan Study. Ann Neurol. 2000;47:145–51.
24. Case NF, Charlton A, Zwiers A, et al. Cerebral amyloid angiopathy is associated with executive dysfunction and mild cognitive impairment. Stroke. 2016;47:2010–6.
25. Amberla K, Waljas M, Tuominen S, et al. Insidious cognitive decline in CADASIL. Stroke. 2004;35:1598–602.
26. Thanvi B, Lo N, Robinson T. Vascular parkinsonism—an important cause of parkinsonism in older people. Age Ageing. 2005;34:114–9.
27. Fuh JL, Wang SJ, Cummings JL. Neuropsychiatric profiles in patients with Alzheimer's disease and vascular dementia. J Neurol Neurosurg Psychiatry. 2005;76:1337–41.
28. Kalimo H, Ruchoux MM, Viitanen M, Kalaria RN. CADASIL: a common form of hereditary arteriopathy causing brain infarcts and dementia. Brain Pathol. 2002;12:371–84.
29. Byram K, Hajj-Ali RA, Calabrese L. CNS vasculitis: an approach to differential diagnosis and management. Curr Rheumatol Rep. 2018;20:37.
30. Gorelick PB, Scuteri A, Black SE, et al. Vascular contributions to cognitive impairment and dementia: a statement for healthcare professionals from the American Heart Association/ American Stroke Association. Stroke. 2011;42:2672–713.
31. Association AP. Diagnostic and statistical manual of mental disorders. BMC Med. 2013;17:133–7.
32. Arvanitakis Z, Capuano AW, Leurgans SE, Bennett DA, Schneider JA. Relation of cerebral vessel disease to Alzheimer's disease dementia and cognitive function in elderly people: a cross-sectional study. Lancet Neurol. 2016;15:934–43.
33. Brainin M, Tuomilehto J, Heiss WD, et al. Post-stroke cognitive decline: an update and perspectives for clinical research. Eur J Neurol. 2015;22:229–38, e213–26.
34. Wardlaw JM, Smith EE, Biessels GJ, et al. Neuroimaging standards for research into small vessel disease and its contribution to ageing and neurodegeneration. Lancet Neurol. 2013;12:822–38.
35. van Straaten EC, Scheltens P, Barkhof F. MRI and CT in the diagnosis of vascular dementia. J Neurol Sci. 2004;226:9–12.
36. Wardlaw JM, Brindle W, Casado AM, et al. A systematic review of the utility of 1.5 versus 3 Tesla magnetic resonance brain imaging in clinical practice and research. Eur Radiol. 2012;22:2295–303.
37. Biesbroek JM, Weaver NA, Biessels GJ. Lesion location and cognitive impact of cerebral small vessel disease. Clin Sci (Lond). 2017;131:715–28.
38. Allen LM, Hasso AN, Handwerker J, Farid H. Sequence-specific MR imaging findings that are useful in dating ischemic stroke. Radiographics. 2012;32:1285–97; discussion 1297–9.
39. Srinivasan A, Goyal M, Al Azri F, Lum C. State-of-the-art imaging of acute stroke. Radiographics. 2006;26(Suppl 1):S75–95.
40. Levine DA, Galecki AT, Langa KM, et al. Trajectory of cognitive decline after incident stroke. JAMA. 2015;314:41–51.
41. Hachinski V, Iadecola C, Petersen RC, et al. National Institute of Neurological Disorders and Stroke-Canadian Stroke Network vascular cognitive impairment harmonization standards. Stroke. 2006;37:2220–41.
42. Boon A, Lodder J, Heuts-van Raak L, Kessels F. Silent brain infarcts in 755 consecutive patients with a first-ever supratentorial ischemic stroke. Relationship with index-stroke subtype, vascular risk factors, and mortality. Stroke. 1994;25:2384–90.
43. Fanning JP, Wong AA, Fraser JF. The epidemiology of silent brain infarction: a systematic review of population-based cohorts. BMC Med. 2014;12:119.

44. Wright CB, Festa JR, Paik MC, et al. White matter hyperintensities and subclinical infarction: associations with psychomotor speed and cognitive flexibility. Stroke. 2008;39:800–5.
45. Liebetrau M, Steen B, Hamann GF, Skoog I. Silent and symptomatic infarcts on cranial computerized tomography in relation to dementia and mortality: a population-based study in 85-year-old subjects. Stroke. 2004;35:1816–20.
46. Zhao L, Biesbroek JM, Shi L, et al. Strategic infarct location for post-stroke cognitive impairment: a multivariate lesion-symptom mapping study. J Cereb Blood Flow Metab. 2018;38:1299–311.
47. Hachinski VC, Potter P, Merskey H. Leuko-araiosis. Arch Neurol. 1987;44:21–3.
48. de Leeuw FE, de Groot JC, Achten E, et al. Prevalence of cerebral white matter lesions in elderly people: a population based magnetic resonance imaging study. The Rotterdam Scan Study. J Neurol Neurosurg Psychiatry. 2001;70:9–14.
49. Brickman AM, Schupf N, Manly JJ, et al. Brain morphology in older African Americans, Caribbean Hispanics, and whites from northern Manhattan. Arch Neurol. 2008;65:1053–61.
50. Morris Z, Whiteley WN, Longstreth WT, et al. Incidental findings on brain magnetic resonance imaging: systematic review and meta-analysis. BMJ. 2009;339:b3016.
51. Chowdhury MH, Nagai A, Bokura H, et al. Age-related changes in white matter lesions, hippocampal atrophy, and cerebral microbleeds in healthy subjects without major cerebrovascular risk factors. J Stroke Cerebrovasc Dis. 2011;20:302–9.
52. Tomimoto H. Subcortical vascular dementia. Neurosci Res. 2011;71:193–9.
53. Kanekar S, Poot JD. Neuroimaging of vascular dementia. Radiol Clin N Am. 2014;52:383–401.
54. Charil A, Yousry TA, Rovaris M, et al. MRI and the diagnosis of multiple sclerosis: expanding the concept of "no better explanation". Lancet Neurol. 2006;5:841–52.
55. Fazekas F, Chawluk JB, Alavi A, Hurtig HI, Zimmerman RA. MR signal abnormalities at 1.5 T in Alzheimer's dementia and normal aging. AJR Am J Roentgenol. 1987;149:351–6.
56. Fazekas F, Kleinert R, Offenbacher H, et al. Pathologic correlates of incidental MRI white matter signal hyperintensities. Neurology. 1993;43:1683.
57. Haller S, Kovari E, Herrmann FR, et al. Do brain T2/FLAIR white matter hyperintensities correspond to myelin loss in normal aging? A radiologic-neuropathologic correlation study. Acta Neuropathol Commun. 2013;1:14.
58. Debette S, Bombois S, Bruandet A, et al. Subcortical hyperintensities are associated with cognitive decline in patients with mild cognitive impairment. Stroke. 2007;38:2924–30.
59. de Groot JC, de Leeuw FE, Oudkerk M, et al. Cerebral white matter lesions and depressive symptoms in elderly adults. Arch Gen Psychiatry. 2000;57:1071–6.
60. Yousry TA, Seelos K, Mayer M, et al. Characteristic MR lesion pattern and correlation of T1 and T2 lesion volume with neurologic and neuropsychological findings in cerebral autosomal dominant arteriopathy with subcortical infarcts and leukoencephalopathy (CADASIL). AJNR Am J Neuroradiol. 1999;20:91–100.
61. Scheltens P, Barkhof F, Leys D, et al. A semiquantitative rating scale for the assessment of signal hyperintensities on magnetic resonance imaging. J Neurol Sci. 1993;114:7–12.
62. Inzitari D, Simoni M, Pracucci G, et al. Risk of rapid global functional decline in elderly patients with severe cerebral age-related white matter changes: the LADIS study. Arch Intern Med. 2007;167:81–8.
63. Inzitari D, Pracucci G, Poggesi A, et al. Changes in white matter as determinant of global functional decline in older independent outpatients: three year follow-up of LADIS (leuko-araiosis and disability) study cohort. BMJ. 2009;339:b2477.
64. Godin O, Tzourio C, Rouaud O, et al. Joint effect of white matter lesions and hippocampal volumes on severity of cognitive decline: the 3C-Dijon MRI study. J Alzheimers Dis. 2010;20:453–63.
65. Vemuri P, Lesnick TG, Przybelski SA, et al. Vascular and amyloid pathologies are independent predictors of cognitive decline in normal elderly. Brain. 2015;138:761–71.
66. Lampe L, Kharabian-Masouleh S, Kynast J, et al. Lesion location matters: the relationships between white matter hyperintensities on cognition in the healthy elderly. J Cereb Blood Flow Metab. 2017;39:36–43.

67. Knopman DS, Griswold ME, Lirette ST, et al. Vascular imaging abnormalities and cognition. Stroke. 2015;46:433–40.
68. Au R, Massaro JM, Wolf PA, et al. Association of white matter hyperintensity volume with decreased cognitive functioning. Arch Neurol. 2006;63:246.
69. Camarda C, Torelli P, Pipia C, et al. Association between atrophy of the caudate nuclei, global brain atrophy, cerebral small vessel disease and mild parkinsonian signs in neurologically and cognitively healthy subjects aged 45-84 years: a crosssectional study. Curr Alzheimer Res. 2018;15:1013–26.
70. Willey Joshua Z, Moon Yeseon P, Dhamoon Mandip S, et al. Regional subclinical cerebrovascular disease is associated with balance in an elderly multi-ethnic population. Neuroepidemiology. 2018;51:57–63.
71. Boone KB, Miller BL, Lesser IM, et al. Neuropsychological correlates of white-matter lesions in healthy elderly subjects. A threshold effect. Arch Neurol. 1992;49:549–54.
72. van Straaten EC, Scheltens P, Knol DL, et al. Operational definitions for the NINDS-AIREN criteria for vascular dementia: an interobserver study. Stroke. 2003;34:1907–12.
73. Marks P. Cerebral ischemia and infarction. In: Magnetic resonance imaging of the brain and spine, vol. 1. Philadelphia, PA: Lippincott Williams & Wilkins; 2002. p. 919–79.
74. Wright CB, Dong C, Perez EJ, et al. Subclinical cerebrovascular disease increases the risk of incident stroke and mortality: the northern Manhattan study. J Am Heart Assoc. 2017;6:e004069.
75. Caunca MR, De Leon-Benedetti A, Latour L, Leigh R, Wright CB. Neuroimaging of cerebral small vessel disease and age-related cognitive changes. Front Aging Neurosci. 2019;11:145.
76. Knopman DS, Penman AD, Catellier DJ, et al. Vascular risk factors and longitudinal changes on brain MRI: the ARIC study. Neurology. 2011;76:1879–85.
77. Viswanathan A, Godin O, Jouvent E, et al. Impact of MRI markers in subcortical vascular dementia: a multi-modal analysis in CADASIL. Neurobiol Aging. 2010;31:1629–36.
78. Koga H, Takashima Y, Murakawa R, et al. Cognitive consequences of multiple lacunes and Leukoaraiosis as vascular cognitive impairment in community-dwelling elderly individuals. J Stroke Cerebrovasc Dis. 2009;18:32–7.
79. Vermeer SE, Prins ND, den Heijer T, et al. Silent brain infarcts and the risk of dementia and cognitive decline. N Engl J Med. 2003;348:1215–22.
80. Vital C, Julien J. Expanding lacunae causing triventricular hydrocephalus. J Neurosurg. 2000;93:155–6.
81. De Guio F, Jouvent E, Biessels GJ, et al. Reproducibility and variability of quantitative magnetic resonance imaging markers in cerebral small vessel disease. J Cereb Blood Flow Metab. 2016;36:1319–37.
82. Ramirez J, Berezuk C, McNeely AA, et al. Imaging the perivascular space as a potential biomarker of neurovascular and neurodegenerative diseases. Cell Mol Neurobiol. 2016;36:289–99.
83. Adams HHH, Hilal S, Schwingenschuh P, et al. A priori collaboration in population imaging: the uniform neuro-imaging of Virchow-Robin spaces enlargement consortium. Alzheimer's Dement Diagn Assess Dis Monit. 2015;1:513–20.
84. Gutierrez J, Elkind MSV, Cheung K, et al. Pulsatile and steady components of blood pressure and subclinical cerebrovascular disease. J Hypertens. 2015;33:2115–22.
85. Yao M, Zhu Y-C, Soumaré A, et al. Hippocampal perivascular spaces are related to aging and blood pressure but not to cognition. Neurobiol Aging. 2014;35:2118–25.
86. Yakushiji Y, Charidimou A, Hara M, et al. Topography and associations of perivascular spaces in healthy adults: the Kashima scan study. Neurology. 2014;83:2116–23.
87. MacLullich AMJ. Enlarged perivascular spaces are associated with cognitive function in healthy elderly men. J Neurol Neurosurg Psychiatry. 2004;75:1519–23.
88. Ding J, Sigurðsson S, Jónsson PV, et al. Large perivascular spaces visible on magnetic resonance imaging, cerebral small vessel disease progression, and risk of dementia. JAMA Neurol. 2017;74:1105.

89. Adachi M, Hosoya T, Haku T, Yamaguchi K. Dilated Virchow-Robin spaces: MRI pathological study. Neuroradiology. 1998;40:27–31.
90. Greenberg SM, Vernooij MW, Cordonnier C, et al. Cerebral microbleeds: a guide to detection and interpretation. Lancet Neurol. 2009;8:165–74.
91. Roob G, Schmidt R, Kapeller P, et al. MRI evidence of past cerebral microbleeds in a healthy elderly population. Neurology. 1999;52:991.
92. Ding J, Sigurðsson S, Jónsson PV, et al. Space and location of cerebral microbleeds, cognitive decline, and dementia in the community. Neurology. 2017;88:2089–97.
93. Graff-Radford J, Simino J, Kantarci K, et al. Neuroimaging correlates of cerebral microbleeds. Stroke. 2017;48:2964–72.
94. van Leijsen EMC, van Uden IWM, Ghafoorian M, et al. Nonlinear temporal dynamics of cerebral small vessel disease. Neurology. 2017;89:1569–77.
95. Mittal S, Wu Z, Neelavalli J, Haacke EM. Susceptibility-weighted imaging: technical aspects and clinical applications, part 2. Am J Neuroradiol. 2009;30:232–52.
96. Scheid R, Ott DV, Roth H, Schroeter ML, von Cramon DY. Comparative magnetic resonance imaging at 1.5 and 3 tesla for the evaluation of traumatic microbleeds. J Neurotrauma. 2007;24:1811–6.
97. Stehling C, Wersching H, Kloska SP, et al. Detection of asymptomatic cerebral microbleeds. Acad Radiol. 2008;15:895–900.
98. Barnaure I, Montandon ML, Rodriguez C, et al. Clinicoradiologic correlations of cerebral microbleeds in advanced age. AJNR Am J Neuroradiol. 2017;38:39–45.
99. Romero JR, Preis SR, Beiser A, et al. Risk factors, stroke prevention treatments, and prevalence of cerebral microbleeds in the Framingham heart study. Stroke. 2014;45:1492–4.
100. Poels MM, Vernooij MW, Ikram MA, et al. Prevalence and risk factors of cerebral microbleeds: an update of the Rotterdam scan study. Stroke. 2010;41:S103–6.
101. Vernooij MW, van der Lugt A, Ikram MA, et al. Prevalence and risk factors of cerebral microbleeds: the Rotterdam scan study. Neurology. 2008;70:1208–14.
102. Loehrer E, Ikram M, Akoudad S, et al. Apolipoprotein E-ε4 genotype influences spatial distribution of cerebral microbleeds. Alzheimers Dement. 2013;9:P705.
103. Fagerholm ED, Hellyer PJ, Scott G, Leech R, Sharp DJ. Disconnection of network hubs and cognitive impairment after traumatic brain injury. Brain. 2015;138:1696–709.
104. Poels MMF, Ikram MA, van der Lugt A, et al. Cerebral microbleeds are associated with worse cognitive function: the Rotterdam scan study. Neurology. 2012;78:326–33.
105. Haller S, Vernooij MW, Kuijer JPA, et al. Cerebral microbleeds: imaging and clinical significance. Radiology. 2018;287:11–28.
106. Bobinski M, De Leon M, Wegiel J, et al. The histological validation of post mortem magnetic resonance imaging-determined hippocampal volume in Alzheimer's disease. Neuroscience. 1999;95:721–5.
107. Appelman AP, Exalto LG, Van Der Graaf Y, et al. White matter lesions and brain atrophy: more than shared risk factors? A systematic review. Cerebrovasc Dis. 2009;28:227–42.
108. Aribisala BS, Hernández MCV, Royle NA, et al. Brain atrophy associations with white matter lesions in the ageing brain: the Lothian birth cohort 1936. Eur Radiol. 2013;23:1084–92.
109. Gurol ME, Becker JA, Fotiadis P, et al. Florbetapir-PET to diagnose cerebral amyloid angiopathy: a prospective study. Neurology. 2016;87:2043–9.
110. Heiss WD, Zimmermann-Meinzingen S. PET imaging in the differential diagnosis of vascular dementia. J Neurol Sci. 2012;322:268–73.
111. Klunk WE, Engler H, Nordberg A, et al. Imaging brain amyloid in Alzheimer's disease with Pittsburgh compound-B. Ann Neurol. 2004;55:306–19.
112. Villemagne VL, Ong K, Mulligan RS, et al. Amyloid imaging with (18)F-florbetaben in Alzheimer disease and other dementias. J Nucl Med. 2011;52:1210–7.
113. Cho ME, Kopp JB. Fabry disease in the era of enzyme replacement therapy: a renal perspective. Pediatr Nephrol. 2004;19:583–93.
114. Thiel A, Heiss WD. Imaging of microglia activation in stroke. Stroke. 2011;42:507–12.

115. Radlinska BA, Blunk Y, Leppert IR, et al. Changes in callosal motor fiber integrity after sub-cortical stroke of the pyramidal tract. J Cereb Blood Flow Metab. 2012;32:1515–24.
116. Thiel A, Cechetto DF, Heiss WD, Hachinski V, Whitehead SN. Amyloid burden, neuroin-flammation, and links to cognitive decline after ischemic stroke. Stroke. 2014;45:2825–9.
117. Maillard P, Fletcher E, Lockhart SN, et al. White matter Hyperintensities and their penumbra lie along a continuum of injury in the aging brain. Stroke. 2014;45:1721–6.
118. Seiler S, Fletcher E, Hassan-Ali K, et al. Cerebral tract integrity relates to white matter hyper-intensities, cortex volume, and cognition. Neurobiol Aging. 2018;72:14–22.
119. Cannistraro RJ, Badi M, Eidelman BH, et al. CNS small vessel disease: a clinical review. Neurology. 2019;92:1146–56.
120. Mascalchi M, Salvadori E, Toschi N, et al. DTI-derived indexes of brain WM correlate with cognitive performance in vascular MCI and small-vessel disease. A TBSS study. Brain Imaging Behav. 2019;13:594–602.
121. Baykara E, Gesierich B, Adam R, et al. A novel imaging marker for small vessel disease based on skeletonization of white matter tracts and diffusion histograms. Ann Neurol. 2016;80:581–92.
122. Kim HJ, Im K, Kwon H, et al. Clinical effect of white matter network disruption related to amyloid and small vessel disease. Neurology. 2015;85:63–70.
123. Tuladhar AM, van Dijk E, Zwiers MP, et al. Structural network connectivity and cognition in cerebral small vessel disease. Hum Brain Mapp. 2016;37:300–10.
124. Tuladhar AM, van Uden IW, Rutten-Jacobs LC, et al. Structural network efficiency predicts conversion to dementia. Neurology. 2016;86:1112–9.
125. Ding JR, Ding X, Hua B, et al. Abnormal functional connectivity density in patients with ischemic white matter lesions: an observational study. Medicine (Baltimore). 2016;95:e4625.
126. Ding X, Ding J, Hua B, et al. Abnormal cortical functional activity in patients with ischemic white matter lesions: a resting-state functional magnetic resonance imaging study. Neurosci Lett. 2017;644:10–7.
127. Chen Y, Wang C, Liang H, et al. Resting-state functional magnetic resonance imaging in patients with leukoaraiosis-associated subcortical vascular cognitive impairment: a cross-sectional study. Neurol Res. 2016;38:510–7.
128. Acharya A, Liang X, Tian W, et al. White matter hyperintensities relate to basal ganglia functional connectivity and memory performance in aMCI and SVMCI. Front Neurosci. 2019;13:1204.
129. Langen CD, Zonneveld HI, White T, et al. White matter lesions relate to tract-specific reduc-tions in functional connectivity. Neurobiol Aging. 2017;51:97–103.

Frontotemporal Lobar Degeneration

3

Contents

3.1 Clinicopathological Findings

Frontotemporal lobar degeneration (FTLD) is an umbrella term that encompasses a wide spectrum of clinically, pathologically, and genetically heterogeneous neurodegenerative syndromes that are characterized by progressive changes in behavior, decline in language and executive dysfunction. FTLD is characterized by atrophy and hypometabolism of frontal and anterior temporal lobes with a relative sparing of posterior brain regions.

3.1.1   The Spectrum of FTLD Clinical Presentations

The term "frontotemporal dementia" (FTD) indicates the three main clinical syndromes that are included in the FTLD spectrum, based on the early and predominant symptoms: (1) behavioral variant of frontotemporal dementia (bvFTD), which is characterized by progressive behavioral changes and impairment of executive functions with prevalent atrophy of the frontal lobe (Table 3.1) [1, 2]; (2) non-fluent variant of primary progressive aphasia (nfvPPA), whose hallmarks are effortful, non-fluent speech, agrammatism and limited comprehension of grammatically complex sentences [3, 4] with prevalent atrophy of the left posterior fronto-insular

Table 3.1 International consensus criteria for behavioral variant of frontotemporal dementia

I. Neurodegenerative disease
The following symptom must be present to meet criteria for bvFTD:
Shows progressive deterioration of behavior and/or cognition by observation or history (as provided by a knowledgeable informant).
II. Possible bvFTD
Three of the following behavioral/cognitive symptoms (A–F) must be present to meet criteria. Ascertainment requires that symptoms be persistent or recurrent, rather than single or rare events.

A. Early behavioral disinhibition [one of the following symptoms (A.1–A.3) must be present]:
    A.1. Socially inappropriate behavior.
    A.2. Loss of manners or decorum.
    A.3. Impulsive, rash, or careless actions.

B. Early apathy or inertia [one of the following symptoms (B.1–B.2) must be present]:
    B.1. Apathy.
    B.2. Inertia.

C. Early loss of sympathy or empathy [one of the following symptoms (C.1–C.2) must be present]:
    C.1. Diminished response to other people's needs and feelings.
    C.2. Diminished social interest, interrelatedness, or personal warmth.

D. Early perseverative, stereotype, or compulsive/ritualistic behavior [one of the following symptoms (D.1–D.3) must be present]:
    D.1. Simple repetitive movements.
    D.2. Complex, compulsive, or ritualistic behaviors.
    D.3. Stereotypy of speech.

E. Hyperorality and dietary changes [one of the following symptoms (E.1–E.3) must be present]:
    E.1. Altered food preferences.
    E.2. Binge eating, increased consumption of alcohol or cigarettes.
    E.3. Oral exploration or consumption of inedible objects.

F. Neuropsychological profile: Executive/generation deficits with relative sparing of memory and visuospatial functions [all of the following symptoms (F.1–F.3) must be present]:
    F.1. Deficits in executive tasks.
    F.2. Relative sparing of episodic memory.
    F.3. Relative sparing of visuospatial skills.

Table 3.1 (continued)

III. Probable bvFTD

All of the following symptoms (A–C) must be present to meet criteria:

    A. Meets criteria for possible bvFTD.

    B. Exhibits significant functional decline (by caregiver report or as evidenced by clinical dementia rating scale or functional activities questionnaire scores).

    C. Imaging results consistent with bvFTD [one of the following (C.1–C.2) must be present]:

        C.1. Frontal and/or anterior temporal atrophy on MRI or CT.

        C.2. Frontal and/or anterior temporal hypoperfusion/hypometabolism on PET/SPECT.

IV. Behavioral variant FTD with definite FTLD pathology

Criterion A and either criterion B or C must be present to meet criteria:

    A. Meets criteria for possible or probable bvFTD.

    B. Histopathological evidence of FTLD on biopsy or at post-mortem.

    C. Presence of a known pathogenic mutation.

V. Exclusionary criteria for bvFTD

Criteria A and B must be answered negatively for any bvFTD diagnosis. Criterion C can be positive for possible bvFTD, but must be negative for probable bvFTD:

    A. Pattern of deficits is better accounted for by other non-degenerative nervous system or medical disorders.

    B. Behavioral disturbance is better accounted for by a psychiatric diagnosis.

    C. Biomarkers strongly indicative of AD or other neurodegenerative process.

Reproduced from Rascovsky K, Hodges JR, Knopman D, et al. Sensitivity of revised diagnostic criteria for the behavioral variant of frontotemporal dementia. Brain 2011; 134:2456–2477, by permission of Oxford University Press

Abbreviations: *AD* Alzheimer's disease, *bvFTD* behavioral variant of frontotemporal dementia, *FTLD* frontotemporal lobar degeneration

regions (Table 3.2) [5, 6]; and (3) semantic variant of primary progressive aphasia (svPPA), characterized by confrontation naming difficulty, impaired comprehension of single words, and degraded object knowledge [4, 7] associated with atrophy of the ventral and lateral portions of the anterior temporal lobes bilaterally, although tissue damage is usually more severe in the left hemisphere (Table 3.2) [5, 6]. The FTLD spectrum also displays significant clinical, pathological, and genetic overlap with atypical parkinsonisms such as corticobasal syndrome (CBS) and progressive supranuclear palsy syndrome (PSPs) (see Chap. 4 for further details), as well as with amyotrophic lateral sclerosis (ALS), which can be associated with any of the FTLD clinical syndromes, although the most common association is with bvFTD [8].

3.1.2   Pathology and Genetics

Although the first neuropathological alterations found in cases of dementia with frontotemporal atrophy were intraneuronal inclusions that stained positive for the microtubule-associated protein tau (MAPT) [9, 10], only a fraction of FTLD cases display tau pathology. TAR DNA-binding protein 43 (TDP-43) is the major ubiquitinated

Table 3.2 Diagnostic criteria for the non-fluent and semantic variants of primary progressive aphasia

Non-fluent/agrammatic variant PPA
I. Clinical diagnosis of non-fluent/agrammatic variant PPA
At least one of the following core features must be present:
1. Agrammatism in language production.
2. Effortful, halting speech with inconsistent speech sound errors and distortions (apraxia of speech).
At least 2 of 3 of the following other features must be present:
1. Impaired comprehension of syntactically complex sentences.
2. Spared single-word comprehension.
3. Spared object knowledge.
II. Imaging-supported non-fluent/agrammatic variant diagnosis
Both of the following criteria must be present:
1. Clinical diagnosis of non-fluent/agrammatic variant PPA.
2. Imaging must show one or more of the following results:
a. Predominant left posterior fronto-insular atrophy on MRI; or
b. Predominant left posterior fronto-insular hypoperfusion or hypometabolism on SPECT or PET.
III. Non-fluent/agrammatic variant PPA with definite pathology
Clinical diagnosis (criterion 1 below) and either criterion 2 or 3 must be present:
1. Clinical diagnosis of non-fluent/agrammatic variant PPA.
2. Histopathologic evidence of a specific neurodegenerative pathology (e.g., FTLD-tau, FTLD-TDP, AD, other).
3. Presence of a known pathogenic mutation.
Semantic variant PPA
I. Clinical diagnosis of semantic variant PPA
Both of the following core features must be present:
1. Impaired confrontation naming.
2. Impaired single-word comprehension.
At least three of the following other diagnostic features must be present:
1. Impaired object knowledge, particularly for low-frequency or low-familiarity items.
2. Surface dyslexia or dysgraphia.
3. Spared repetition.
4. Spared speech production (grammar and motor speech).
II. Imaging-supported semantic variant PPA diagnosis
Both of the following criteria must be present:
1. Clinical diagnosis of semantic variant PPA.
2. Imaging must show one or more of the following results:
a. Predominant anterior temporal lobe atrophy.
b. Predominant anterior temporal hypoperfusion or hypometabolism on SPECT or PET.
III. Semantic variant PPA with definite pathology
Clinical diagnosis (criterion 1 below) and either criterion 2 or 3 must be present:
1. Clinical diagnosis of semantic variant PPA.
2. Histopathologic evidence of a specific neurodegenerative pathology (e.g., FTLD-tau, FTLD.TDP, AD, other).
3. Presence of a known pathogenic mutation.

Reproduced from Gorno-Tempini ML, Hillis AE, Weintraub S, et al. Classification of primary progressive aphasia and its variants. Neurology 2011; 76:1006–1014, https://n.neurology.org/, with permission

Abbreviations: *AD* Alzheimer's disease, *FTLD* frontotemporal lobar degeneration, *PPA* primary progressive aphasia

protein associated with tau-negative FTLD [11], and progranulin (GRN) mutations and *C9orf72* expansions are responsible for the majority of TDP-43-positive familial FTLD cases [12, 13]. However, about 5–20% of tau-negative FTLD cases are also TDP-negative, and many of these cases show inclusions of the fused in sarcoma (FUS) protein [8, 14]. Therefore, FTLD spectrum disorders can be divided into three main categories, based on the underlying pathological alterations: (1) tau-associated FTLD (FTLD-tau); (2) TDP-43-associated FTLD (FTLD-TDP); and (3) FUS-associated FTLD (FTLD-FUS). Moreover, several pathological subtypes have been identified, based on the nature and morphology of protein aggregates. Tau exists in two isoforms that result from alternative splicing: a 3-amino-acid sequence repeat form (3R) and a 4-repeat form (4R). The most common tau forms associated with FTD are Pick's disease (3R), corticobasal degeneration (CBD, 4R), and PSP (4R). Four subtypes of FTLD-TDP pathology (A–D) have also been described.

3.2 Neuroimaging

In the last two decades, neuroimaging has contributed to the phenotypic characterization of FTLD syndromes. The most commonly used neuroimaging approaches to assess FTLD are structural magnetic resonance imaging (MRI) and functional molecular techniques, i.e., single photon emission computed tomography (SPECT) and positron emission tomography (PET). The inclusion of typical neuroimaging findings into the revised clinical criteria of bvFTD and PPA variants [2, 4] mirrors the importance of these techniques for an accurate diagnostic approach to these syndromes that might be extended also to other clinical presentations within the FTLD spectrum.

Recent years have also witnessed great advances in the development of novel imaging tools that provide fundamental insights for understanding the pathophysiology of the disease and help in distinguishing FTLD from other neurodegenerative conditions that are in the differential diagnosis, such as Alzheimer's disease (AD). The ability to image amyloid-β (Aβ) and tau pathology using PET ligands may allow easier distinction of FTLD from AD, as well as suggest underlying pathology (i.e., tau versus TDP-43) with greater accuracy. Moreover, alterations in the brain microstructure associated with FTLD can modify water diffusion characteristics, and therefore be measured using diffusion tensor (DT) MRI, whereas early rearrangements in brain function due to FTLD can be detected using functional MRI (fMRI).

3.2.1 Structural Neuroimaging

While computed tomography (CT) can be helpful to exclude other pathology involving the frontal or temporal regions (e.g., a meningioma and vascular disease), MRI is the method of choice to assess the presence and pattern of atrophy in patients with suspected FTD. In this section, gray matter alterations associated with the behavioral and linguistic variants of FTD will be reviewed separately.

3.2.1.1 Behavioral Variant of Frontotemporal Dementia

At structural MRI, bvFTD patients typically present with a combination of medial orbitofrontal, anterior cingulate, insular, and anterior temporal cortical atrophy with an antero-posterior gradient and relative sparing of parietal and occipital lobes [15–19] (Fig. 3.1). This atrophy pattern can be readily appreciated on coronal T1-weighted MRI scans (commonly described as "knife-edge" atrophy due to the severe thinning of cortical gyri) and is often asymmetrical, although commonly bilateral. The medial temporal lobe is also involved, with a greater damage to the amygdala and anterior hippocampi than posterior structures. Brain atrophy in bvFTD also involves several subcortical structures, including the striatum [16, 19, 20], thalamus [19–21], and brainstem [19, 22, 23]. Such pattern is consistent across studies and has shown high sensitivity and specificity in differentiating bvFTD from AD [24], which typically shows an opposite postero-anterior gradient of brain atrophy. The presence of frontal and/or anterior temporal atrophy (as an alternative to hypoperfusion/hypometabolism in the same brain areas) is necessary to make a diagnosis of probable bvFTD according to the current criteria [2], and has shown to provide greatly increased specificity in path-proven cases (up to 95%, compared with 82% when only clinical criteria of possible bvFTD were considered) [25]. Despite such consistency at the group level, great heterogeneity of MRI findings exists among individuals as different cases show variable degrees of hemispheric asymmetry, predominance of frontal versus temporal lobe atrophy and extent of posterior cortical involvement [26]. A large VBM study using cluster analysis suggested that bvFTD may be

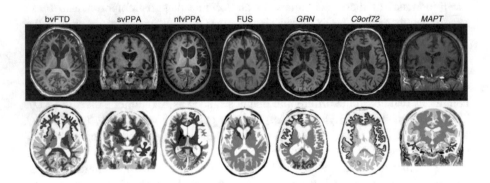

Fig. 3.1 Characteristic patterns of gray matter atrophy (highlighted in red) in different clinical and genetic subtypes of frontotemporal dementia (FTD). Patients with behavioral variant FTD exhibit prominent frontal, insular, and anterior cingulate atrophy. Typical temporal atrophy in semantic variant primary progressive aphasia is asymmetrical (most often left-sided). Patients with non-fluent variant primary progressive aphasia exhibit left frontal and insular atrophy. In patients with underlying RNA-binding protein FUS (FUS) pathology, nucleus caudatus atrophy is pronounced. Patients with *GRN* mutations often exhibit asymmetrical frontotemporoparietal atrophy. Patients with a *C9orf72* repeat expansion present mostly with a generalized symmetrical atrophy. Patients with *MAPT* mutations exhibit marked symmetrical temporal atrophy. *bvFTD* behavioral variant of frontotemporal dementia, *nfvPPA* non-fluent variant primary progressive aphasia, *svPPA* semantic variant primary progressive aphasia. (Reprinted by permission from Springer Nature: Nat Rev. Neurol, Imaging and fluid biomarkers in frontotemporal dementia, Meeter LH, Kaat LD, Rohrer JD, van Swieten JC. © 2017)

divided into four separate neuroanatomical groups, two of which are associated with a prominent frontal atrophy (i.e., frontal dominant and frontotemporal variants) and two with prominent temporal lobe atrophy (i.e., temporal dominant and temporo-frontoparietal subtypes) [27]. Particularly, a right temporal variant of FTD in which the right temporal lobe is the most atrophic region has been associated with clinical features such as behavioral changes, prosopagnosia, and deficits in word-finding and semantic knowledge that show significant overlap with svPPA [27, 28].

This variability in the atrophy patterns among individuals is affected by the great heterogeneity in pathologic and genetic substrates, suggesting distinct anatomical vulnerabilities and informing a clinician's prediction of pathological diagnosis (Fig. 3.1). Within FTLD-tau, Pick's disease is characterized by early severe, asymmetric fronto-insular atrophy that extends into the anterior temporal lobes [29], whereas patients with bvFTD due to CBD show relative preservation of the fronto-insular and temporal structures and greater parietal atrophy [30]. Atrophy of the basal ganglia is more severe in CBD than in PSP [31], whereas cases with PSP pathology show preferential involvement of the brainstem and degeneration of the superior cerebellar peduncle [31, 32]. Patients with FTLD-tau due to mutations on the *MAPT* gene usually display a relatively symmetrical pattern of atrophy involving predominantly the anterior temporal lobes, orbitofrontal cortex, and fornix [33, 34]. Of the four subtypes of FTLD-TDP pathology, types A and B are most commonly observed in bvFTD cases [35]. Type A is usually found in bvFTD patients with *GRN* mutations, who typically show asymmetric atrophy extending into the parietal lobes with relative sparing of the cerebellum [36, 37]. FTLD-TDP type B pathology is often observed in FTD cases with concurrent motor neuron disease (FTD-MND), and is associated with predominant symmetrical atrophy of the frontal lobes and involvement of the insula and the anterior temporal lobe [38]. The *C9orf72* repeat expansion has been associated both with FTLD-TDP type B and, more rarely, with type A pathology or a combination thereof [39–41]. The pattern of atrophy associated with this genetic alteration has only recently been assessed, with some variability across studies. Most studies have found that this genetic abnormality is associated with relatively symmetric patterns of atrophy, mostly in the frontal lobes, although a characteristic spreading to occipital and cerebellar regions has also been described [42–44]. The presence of subcortical—particularly, thalamic—atrophy has been recently reported as a consistent characteristic of *C9orf72*-positive cases [45, 46], with a distinctive involvement of the pulvinar [47]. FTLD-TDP type C is the prevalent underlying pathology of the right temporal variant of bvFTD, representing basically the right-predominant variant of svPPA [48]. Finally, FTLD-FUS is a rare pathological cause of bvFTD, which presents with characteristic severe caudate atrophy [49–51].

Despite the variability of atrophy patterns, visual inspection of regional atrophy may aid the clinician in discriminating between different FTLD subtypes. An a priori classification algorithm based on the presence of a combination of genetic, clinical, and neuroanatomical alterations shown by MRI has been recently applied to a cohort of bvFTD patients with pathological diagnosis, showing a correct inference of underlying pathology in 75 out of 101 patients (Fig. 3.2) [35]. Moreover, several

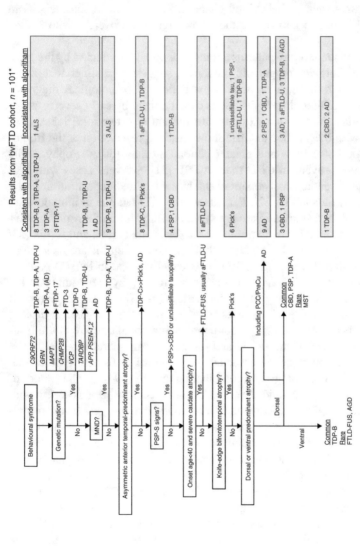

Fig. 3.2 A priori algorithm for pathological prediction in the behavioral variant of frontotemporal dementia (bvFTD). The algorithm is shown on the left, with branches leading to a list of likely pathological diagnoses. On the right are the results from applying the algorithm to the bvFTD cohort, including the numbers of patients whose diagnoses were consistent or inconsistent with the algorithm's prediction. *Sixteen patients could not be fully classified by the algorithm because of lack of imaging. *AD* Alzheimer's disease, *aFTLD-U* atypical FTLD with ubiquitin positive inclusions, *AGD* argyrophilic grain disease, *ALS* amyotrophic lateral sclerosis, *bvFTD* behavioral variant of frontotemporal dementia, *CBD* corticobasal degeneration, *MND* motor neuron disease, *MST* multiple system tauopathy, *PCC* posterior cingulate cortex, *PreCu* precuneus, *PSP* progressive supranuclear palsy, *PSP-S* PSP syndrome, *TDP-U* unclassifiable TDP-43. (Reproduced from Perry DC, Brown JA, Possin KL, et al. Clinicopathological correlations in behavioral variant frontotemporal dementia. Brain 2017; 140:3329–3345, by permission of Oxford University Press)

studies have assessed the discriminatory power of atrophy patterns to distinguish FTLD from AD. In fact, FTLD is associated with greater atrophy in the frontal, insular, anterior cingulate cortices, and striatum, whereas AD is characterized by a more severe damage to the posterior cingulate, precuneus, and occipital regions [52]. The presence of either severe frontal atrophy or asymmetry was found to be highly diagnostic of bvFTD compared with AD and vascular dementia cases [53]. In a study assessing patients with pathologically confirmed diagnosis, atrophy of the anterior, inferior, and lateral temporal lobes, antero-posterior gradient and hemispheric asymmetry of atrophy were each at least 85% specific for FTLD versus AD pathology [54]. Studies comparing bvFTD with both typical and atypical AD phenotypes (i.e., early-onset AD, or AD cases with prominent behavioral or language deficits) have suggested that, independent of clinical phenotype, a cortical thinning of the anterior temporal and frontal lobes is indicative of FTLD, whereas atrophy of the posterior cingulate gyrus, parietal lobe, and frontal pole indicates AD pathology [55–57].

It should be considered that in early stages of bvFTD structural imaging is often normal. Although many patients will progress to show frontotemporal atrophy, a small number of cases appear to clinically progress slowly in terms of behavioral symptoms with little or no atrophy on longitudinal MR scanning [58, 59]. These subjects have been referred to as having a bvFTD "phenocopy syndrome," as some of these subjects may not have an underlying FTLD pathology and instead might represent a psychiatric phenocopy [60].

3.2.1.2 Primary Progressive Aphasia

The non-fluent variant of PPA is characteristically associated with left anterior perisylvian atrophy, involving the inferior frontal gyrus (including Broca's area), premotor, dorsolateral prefrontal, and anterior insular cortex (Fig. 3.1) [5, 61]. As language deficits worsen, ipsilateral anterior frontal, lateral temporal, and anterior parietal lobes show increasing atrophy, and posterior frontal and temporal lobe structures in the right hemisphere also get involved (Fig. 3.3) [6, 61]. Moreover, bilateral atrophy of the basal ganglia, thalamus, and amygdala has been observed in nfvPPA patients [5, 62]. Although left hippocampal atrophy has also been reported, this is typically less severe relative to AD patients [63].

Similar to nfvPPA, patients with svPPA also show predominant involvement of the left hemisphere, with typical atrophy of the anterior temporal lobe (i.e., temporal pole) mainly affecting the lateral and ventral temporal surfaces, as well as the anterior hippocampus, amygdala, and fusiform gyrus (Fig. 3.1) [5, 15, 64, 65]. Semantic patients may have hippocampal atrophy that is at least as severe as that seen in AD patients, although predominantly located in the anterior regions [63, 65, 66]. Temporal lobe atrophy is also mainly inferior, often with a severe involvement of the fusiform gyrus and a relative sparing of the superior temporal gyrus [67, 68]. Although the most common variant of svPPA displays left greater than right temporal lobe atrophy, the opposite pattern can be observed less frequently in cases showing significant overlap with the right temporal variant of bvFTD [69]. As the disease progresses, greater atrophy of posterior and superior temporal, frontal

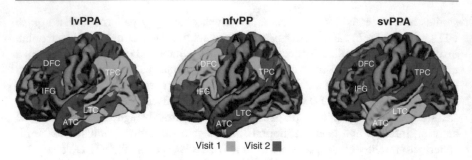

Fig. 3.3 Progression of cortical thinning in the left hemisphere by primary progressive aphasia subtype. Areas of significant cortical thinning in the left hemisphere at baseline (green) and 2 years later (blue) for each of the primary progressive aphasia variants. *ATC* anterior temporal cortex, *DFC* dorsal frontal cortex, *IFG* inferior frontal gyrus, *LTC* lateral temporal cortex, *lvPPA* logopenic primary progressive aphasia subtype, *nfvPPA* non-fluent/agrammatic primary progressive aphasia subtype, *svPPA* semantic primary progressive aphasia subtype, *TPC* temporoparietal cortex. (Reproduced from Rogalski E, Cobia D, Harrison TM, et al. Progression of language decline and cortical atrophy in subtypes of primary progressive aphasia. Neurology 2011; 76:1804–1810, https://n.neurology.org/, with permission)

(orbitofrontal, inferior frontal, and cingulate gyri), and insular regions can be detected (Fig. 3.3) [6, 70].

In a similar way to bvFTD, the assessment of atrophy patterns on conventional MRI has been included in the current diagnostic criteria of PPA clinical variants [4], as a possible method to make an "imaging-supported" diagnosis (Table 3.2). Although there is no absolute association between each PPA variant and a single pathological entity, nfvPPA is mainly associated with FTLD-tau [71–74], whereas most svPPA cases show underlying FTLD-TDP pathology [71, 73–75]. A third variant of PPA, the logopenic variant (lvPPA) is mainly caused by AD, rather than FTLD pathology (see Chap. 1 and related figures for further details) [73, 76, 77], but its distinction from nfvPPA may be challenging based on clinical features alone [78]. A recent clinicopathological review [73] has highlighted the importance of an imaging-supported diagnosis to increase the correspondence between each PPA clinical variant and a highly typical (83–100%) pathological correlate. Atrophy of the temporoparietal junction has been indicated as a key element to discriminate between nfvPPA and lvPPA cases at an individual patient level [78], as this is characteristically involved at the early stages of lvPPA [79]. Similarly, differential atrophy of the left temporal pole and pars opercularis of the inferior frontal gyrus was shown to aid in the discrimination between nfvPPA and svPPA [80]. However, initial distinctive neuroanatomical features can be very subtle in the early phase of the disease or may be lost as degeneration progresses and converges over time (Fig. 3.3) [6, 61]. It has also been suggested that specific neuroimaging features may suggest the presence of "atypical" pathology in sporadic presentations of PPA (e.g., frontal cortical atrophy in svPPA cases with FTLD-tau, and absence of subcortical atrophy in nfvPPA cases with FTLD-TDP) [73], and characteristic frontal atrophy has been shown for right hemispheric svPPA patients with FTLD-tau pathology due to MAPT

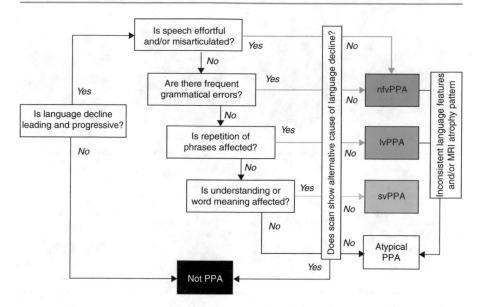

Fig. 3.4 An algorithm for diagnosis of primary progressive aphasia syndromes. Brain imaging (wherever feasible, MRI) is essential to rule out brain tumors and other non-degenerative pathologies that can occasionally present with progressive aphasia, and also has an important "positive" role in corroborating the neuroanatomical diagnosis. *lvPPA* logopenic primary progressive aphasia subtype, *nfvPPA* non-fluent/agrammatic primary progressive aphasia subtype, *PPA* primary progressive aphasia, *svPPA* semantic primary progressive aphasia subtype. (Adapted from Marshall CR, Hardy CJD, Volkmer A, et al. Primary progressive aphasia: a clinical approach. J Neurol 2018; 265:1474–1490, an article distributed under the terms of the Creative Commons Attribution 4.0 International License)

mutations, compared with FTLD-TDP cases with a similar clinical presentation [69]. See Fig. 3.4 for a schematic representation of the diagnostic algorithm of PPA variants based on the combination of cognitive and MRI features.

3.2.2 Molecular Imaging

3.2.2.1 SPECT and PET Imaging

SPECT or PET scans of bvFTD cases typically identify patterns of hypoperfusion or hypometabolism—respectively—in frontal, insular, and anterior temporal regions (Fig. 3.5) [81–83]. The most severely impaired regions are the medial frontal cortex, the frontolateral, and anterior temporal cortices. Such characteristic pattern of hypoperfusion or hypometabolism on SPECT or PET scans has demonstrated to greatly increase the sensitivity of detecting bvFTD, compared with clinical diagnosis alone [84]. In fact, SPECT or PET scans represent a valid alternative to structural MRI to make a diagnosis of probable bvFTD according to the current criteria [2], possibly indicating frontal and temporal alterations that precede the development of gray

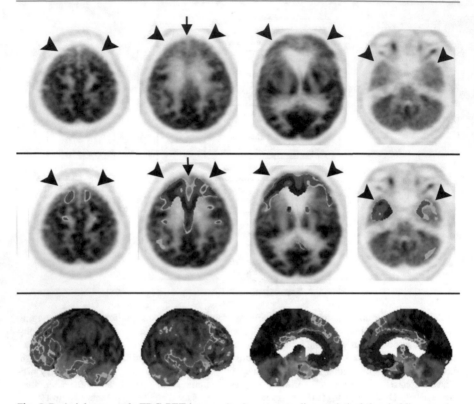

Fig. 3.5 Axial gray-scale FDG-PET images (top), corresponding statistical thresholding overlay images (middle), and 3D-Statistical Surface Projections (SSP) images (bottom) (left to right: left lateral, right lateral, left medial, and right medial views) show moderate bilateral frontal and anterior temporal lobe hypometabolism (arrowheads) in a pattern that is characteristic of behavioral variant of frontotemporal dementia. There is anterior cingulate gyral hypometabolism (arrows) as well as relatively preserved posterior cingulate–precuneus metabolism; findings that are best appreciated on the 3D SSP images. Blue = −2 SDs, purple = −3 SDs. (Reproduced with permission from Brown RKJ, Bohnen NI, Wong KK, et al. Brain PET in suspected dementia: Patterns of altered FDG metabolism. RadioGraphics. 2014;34:684–701)

matter atrophy [85]. However, metabolic abnormalities are not limited to these regions. As dementia progresses, the severity and extent of perfusion and metabolic impairment also increases and starts to involve other associative regions [86].

The predominantly frontal pattern of functional impairment, associated with a relative sparing of posterior brain regions, usually allows a clear distinction between bvFTD patients and those with AD [53, 83, 87–90]. Using an anterior–posterior cerebral blood flow SPECT ratio (medial superior frontal gyrus/medial temporal lobes), patients with clinical bvFTD were successfully distinguished from AD patients with high sensitivity and specificity, both when early-onset and late-onset AD cases were considered [87]. A reduction of frontal blood flow has also been indicated as a marker of pathologically confirmed FTLD when compared with proven AD cases (sensitivity 80%, specificity 65%), particularly when this is not associated with parietal abnormalities (sensitivity 80%, specificity 81%) [91]. However, an overlap of abnormalities between these two conditions exists since AD can involve frontal regions and FTLD may not spare the temporoparietal cortex [92]. In recent years, the use of PET with ^{18}F-fluorodeoxyglucose (FDG-PET) has de facto replaced SPECT as the main technique to assess functional alterations of neurodegenerative diseases in the clinical context, both by visual inspection and especially by quantitative assessment [93]. A pattern of (often asymmetrical) hypo-metabolism involving the orbitofrontal, dorsolateral, medial prefrontal, and anterior temporal cortices, as well as the basal ganglia, has shown to differentiate patients with bvFTD from individuals with other dementia types and healthy controls with a sensitivity and specificity ranging from 80% to 95% [85, 86, 93–95].

Patterns of focal hypometabolism vary between clinical variants of PPA, mirror-ing the structural changes described in the previous sections and providing similar suggestions for the differential diagnosis (Fig. 3.5) (see also Chap. 1, Fig. 1.7). In nfvPPA patients, functional deficits of the left frontal opercular regions have been reported consistently [96–99], often associated with an involvement of bilateral caudate nuclei and thalami (Fig. 3.5) [99]. A PET study of non-fluent patients dem-onstrated that a pattern of bilateral temporoparietal involvement is predictive of AD pathology, while a unilateral (left) temporoparietal cortex hypometabolism/perfu-sion was seen in cases with FTLD pathology; on the contrary, a bilaterally normal temporoparietal cortical perfusion or metabolism was predictive of FTLD pathol-ogy [100]. In patients with svPPA, FDG-PET studies have showed asymmetrical hypometabolism of the temporal lobes, more marked on the left side (Fig. 3.5) [96, 101, 102]. A study comparing svPPA and very early AD patients using structural MRI and FDG-PET revealed hippocampal atrophy and hypometabolism in both groups; however, AD patients showed a strikingly reduced metabolism of the poste-rior cingulate cortex, which was not detected in those with svPPA [101].

Regarding different genetic forms of FTD, *GRN* mutation carriers typically dis-play asymmetrical hypometabolism in frontal and temporal brain regions [103, 104], *C9orf72* expansions are associated with hypometabolism in the limbic sys-tem, basal ganglia, and thalamus [105], whereas *MAPT* mutations are associated with hypometabolism in the medial temporal lobe and the frontal and parietal corti-ces [106] (Fig. 3.6).

Consistent with the diagnostic algorithm previously described for the distinction between AD and other dementias (see Chap. 1, Fig. 1.1), the pattern of hypometabo-lism observed on imaging might be particularly useful when, following clinical assessment and structural imaging, AD is not the single most probable or suspected diagnosis. In these cases, the use of FDG-PET might be conclusive for a specific form of non-AD dementia (e.g., an FTLD clinical variant), without any evident need for further testing of amyloid pathology by means of other PET and/or CSF bio-markers [107].

3.2.2.2 Amyloid PET

In the last two decades, PET imaging tracers have been developed to demonstrate the presence of abnormal amyloid aggregates in the central nervous system,

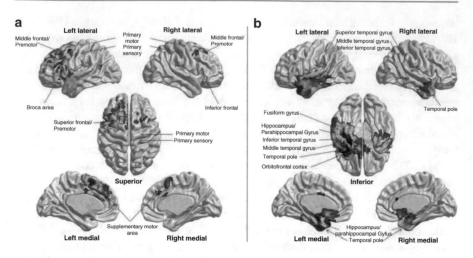

Fig. 3.6 Surface projections of typical patterns of hypometabolism in non-fluent/agrammatic variant primary progressive aphasia (**a**) and semantic variant primary progressive aphasia (**b**). (Reproduced from Botha H, Josephs KA. Primary Progressive Aphasias and Apraxia of Speech. Continuum (Minneap Minn) 2019; 25 (1): 101–127, https://journals.lww.com/continuum/pages/default.aspx, with permission)

allowing to visualize neuropathology in vivo. Amyloid imaging is particularly helpful in distinguishing FTLD, which is not associated with amyloid deposition, from AD, in which amyloid plaques are a characteristic pathologic hallmark (Fig. 3.7) (see also Chap. 1, Fig. 1.9). In fact, low cortical ^{11}C-Pittsburgh compound B (PIB), ^{18}F-florbetaben, or ^{18}F-florbetapir uptake has been observed in patients with bvFTD [108–114], assisting the differentiation of AD from FTD with relatively high sensitivity and specificity [102, 110, 112, 114]. In a large study assessing 62 AD and 45 FTD patients, ^{11}C-PIB scans were positive in 87% of AD cases and 16% of FTD cases, with higher sensitivity for AD compared with FDG-PET (89% versus 77%) and similar specificity (83% versus 84%) [112]. Amyloid PET is particularly useful for the differentiation of lvPPA patients from other PPA syndromes, as the former usually have underlying AD pathology and therefore amyloid tracer retention (Fig. 3.7) (see also Chap. 1, Fig. 1.9), with a pattern that is indistinguishable from that of typical AD [96, 111, 115]. It has to be noted that patient classification in most of these studies was based on clinical diagnosis as histopathological confirmation was available only in a minority of cases [112]; therefore, the FTD cases that were found positive at amyloid imaging might be due to either misclassification or comorbid FTLD and AD pathology. The co-occurrence of FTLD and AD pathology becomes more likely with increasing age, so the presence of a positive amyloid scan in a patient older than 70 years old with a clinical suspect of FTD [116, 117] is less helpful than in younger individuals, particularly as amyloid positivity can be observed even decades prior to the development of AD symptoms [118]. Therefore, amyloid imaging is fundamental for a correct diagnostic process in early-onset

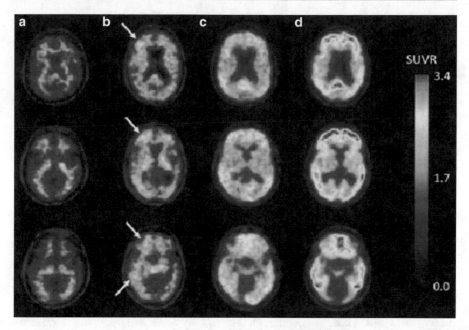

Fig. 3.7 Representative examples of ^{11}C-labeled Pittsburgh Compound B (PIB)-PET scanning. (**a**) PIB-PET image of a negative scan. (**b**) Image of the logopenic case who had a positive scan. Arrows indicate the cortical regions with a PIB-standardized uptake value ratio higher than 1.50. (**c, d**) Images show positive scans of logopenic and typical Alzheimer's disease cases, respectively. *SUVR* standardized uptake value ratio. (Reproduced from Leyton CE, Villemagne VL, Savage S, et al. Subtypes of progressive aphasia: application of the International Consensus Criteria and validation using beta-amyloid imaging. Brain 2011; 134:3030–3043, by permission of Oxford University Press)

dementia, but its positivity in older patients does not rule out an FTLD etiology. Moreover, amyloid PET does not help to differentiate between FTLD-tau and FTLD-TDP pathologies.

3.2.2.3 Tau PET

PET ligands selective for tau pathology have been recently developed, although mostly applied to the study of AD-related tauopathy [119]. However, this technique has clear potential for aiding the differential diagnosis between pathological subtypes of FTLD and quantifying tau burden in primary tauopathies (such as PSP and CBS), possibly providing important surrogate outcome measures to evaluate the efficacy of tau-targeted therapy. To date, only few tau PET studies have been performed in FTLD. ^{18}F-flortaucipir (formerly known as ^{18}F-AV-1451), ^{18}F-THK, and ^{11}C-PBB3 tracers have been used in single cases or small cohorts of patients with PSP or CBS, showing the expected regional distribution of tau pathology of these clinical presentations with good discrimination from healthy individuals [120–125], typical AD [122, 124], and Parkinson's disease [123] patients. However, considering that the target regions of PSP and CBS pathological alterations often coincide with areas of off-target binding of tau PET tracers—particularly, ^{18}F-flortaucipir—to MAO-B enzyme in the basal ganglia, there is a large overlap in the pattern of tracer binding in these regions across different diagnostic groups [123, 125]. Moreover, both ^{18}F-flortaucipir and ^{18}F-THK ligands have shown off-target binding to protein deposits other than tau. For instance, high binding of both tracers within the anterior temporal lobes has been observed in patients with a clinical diagnosis of svPPA, an FTLD syndrome which is not primarily associated with the presence of tau, but rather TDP-43 pathology [126, 127]. Therefore, although tau PET represents a promising advance in the imaging of neurodegeneration, the development of more specific tracers with post-mortem validation is needed to allow its use in the clinical field for improving differential diagnosis and elucidating the evolution of tau deposits in the brain of FTLD patients.

3.2.3 Advanced MRI Techniques

3.2.3.1 Diffusion Tensor MRI
Abnormalities of the white matter are considered as key neuropathological underpinnings of FTLD [128, 129], although they usually occur at a microstructural level that can be detected only using advanced MRI techniques (i.e., diffusion tensor [DT] MRI). Several studies have explored DT MRI alterations in FTLD presentations, providing insights that are summarized in the following paragraphs relative to bvFTD and PPA presentations.

Although white matter abnormalities in FTLD are mostly microstructural—therefore, detectable only after post-processing of raw imaging data—an exception is constituted by the white matter hyperintensities that are characteristic of *GRN* mutations; these are macroscopically detectable on T2-weighted sequences, although they occur only in a subset of patients [130, 131]. Neuropathological studies have suggested that these white matter hyperintensities might not be vascular in origin, but rather associated with prominent microglial activation [132].

In bvFTD, several studies found DT MRI abnormalities in white matter tracts located in the frontal lobes, such as the anterior cingulum, genu of the corpus callosum, and superior longitudinal fasciculus (SLF), and in those tracts passing through the temporal lobes, such as the uncinate, inferior longitudinal fasciculus (ILF), and inferior fronto-occipital fasciculus (IFOF) [133–136]. Diffusivity abnormalities have also been reported in more posterior white matter regions, including the posterior SLF and cingulum [133, 135]. The cingulum and uncinate fasciculus are particularly affected in bvFTD patients with a *MAPT* mutation [137], whereas greater involvement of the IFOF and distinctive DT MRI abnormalities in the corticospinal tracts, thalamic radiations, and superior cerebellar peduncles have been reported in *C9orf72* mutation carriers [42, 45]. When neuroimaging data of FTLD cases with either tau or TDP-43 pathology were directly compared, FTLD-tau showed significantly greater WM degeneration relative to FTLD-TDP [138, 139], consistent with greater inclusion severity at autopsy [138], supporting a central role for DT MRI to allow an in vivo discrimination of underlying pathology in FTLD.

DT MRI has also proven to potentially improve the diagnostic differentiation between bvFTD and AD. In several studies, when compared with AD, bvFTD patients have shown greater disruption of widespread anterior WM regions, namely the genu of the corpus callosum, IFOF, cingulum, uncinate, and frontal corona radiata [57, 135, 140]. In particular, WM damage of the uncinate fasciculus has been suggested as a key predictor to distinguish bvFTD from early-onset AD clinical presentations [57]. By contrast, AD patients generally did not show areas of significant WM damage relative to FTD patients [135, 140], thus suggesting that WM injury might be more prominent in bvFTD than in AD.

The non-fluent variant of PPA is characterized by a prominent involvement of the left SLF [133, 134, 136, 141–143], although a significant involvement of the corpus callosum, cingulum bundle, external capsule, several regions of the prefrontal and orbitofrontal white matter, parietotemporal white matter, and temporal regions has also been found [133, 142]. By contrast, ventral tracts connecting the temporal lobe with occipital and orbitofrontal regions (i.e., the ILF and uncinate fasciculi) are relatively spared in nfvPPA (Fig. 3.8) [134, 141]. In patients with prominent apraxia of speech, white matter connections within the frontal lobe and in fronto-striatal circuits show prominent damage [144]. The frontal aslant tract, which connects Broca's area to the anterior supplementary motor regions, is particularly vulnerable in nfvPPA with apraxia of speech [145].

In svPPA, white matter microstructural abnormalities have been identified in the major inferior and superior connections of the left temporal lobe, mirroring the severe atrophy affecting the same regions, i.e., the ILF, IFOF, and uncinate fasciculus of the ventral stream, and also the temporoparietal component of the SLF of the dorsal stream [133, 134, 136, 141, 142, 146, 147]. By contrast, the frontoparietal portions of the SLF and the frontal speech network are relatively spared, consistent with the sparing of phonological and grammatical knowledge in these patients [80, 141, 148].

Damage to the frontal aslant tract and genu of the corpus callosum has been suggested to help in the discrimination of nfvPPA cases from lvPPA at an individual patient level [78], whereas a greater involvement of tracts of the ventral stream (i.e., the uncinate and ILF) has proven to indicate an svPPA diagnosis when nfvPPA is in the differential [80].

3.2.3.2 Functional MRI

Functional MRI (fMRI) is likely to detect alterations in brain function that may be present very early in the course of FTLD. In particular, resting state (RS) fMRI allows the characterization of low-frequency, spontaneous fluctuations of blood oxygenation level-dependent (BOLD) signal across the brain that are organized into distinct, tightly correlated functional-anatomic networks, some of which are typically disrupted in these conditions.

Several studies which have explored the RS functional connectivity in patients with bvFTD [149–152] demonstrated an altered connectivity of the salience

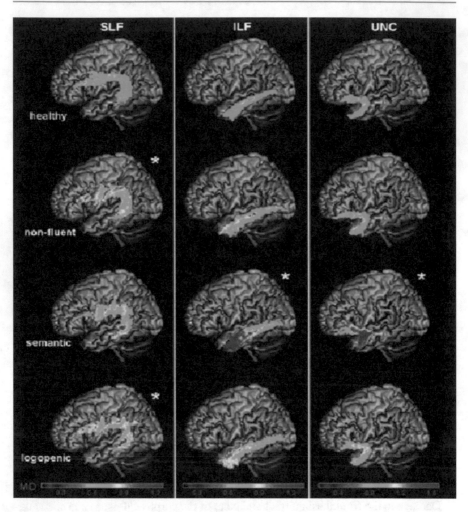

Fig. 3.8 Mean diffusivity values of each group in the probability maps for left superior longitudinal fasciculus (SLF), inferior longitudinal fasciculus (ILF), uncinate fasciculus (UNC), overlaid on a standard MNI brain. Only voxels that are in common in at least 20% of the subjects in each group were included in the probability maps. Asterisk denotes significantly different relative to normal controls at $P < 0.05$. The chromatic scale represents average mean diffusivity values ranging from lower (violet–blue) to higher values (yellow–red). MD is measured in $mm^2/s \times 10^{-3}$. *MD* mean diffusivity. (Reproduced from Galantucci S, Tartaglia MC, Wilson SM, et al. White matter damage in primary progressive aphasias: a diffusion tensor tractography study. Brain 2011; 134:3011–3029, by permission of Oxford University Press)

network, which is involved in emotional processing, behavior and interpersonal experiences [153], most notably in the frontal and anterior insula, mid-cingulate and numerous subcortical, limbic, and brainstem regions. A co-occurrent increased functional connectivity of the default-mode network (DMN) has also been reported in bvFTD patients [149, 150], which contrasts with the disrupted connectivity of the

DMN that is typically found in AD patients [149]. A combination of salience network and DMN connectivity scores was able to classify healthy subjects, AD patients, and bvFTD patients with a 92% accuracy, and to separate AD and bvFTD patients with a 100% accuracy [149]. Network analysis based on graph theoretical models was also applied to RS fMRI data from patients with bvFTD [154], demonstrating global and local functional network abnormalities that were located in structures known to harbor the neuropathological changes of bvFTD, such as the frontotemporal lobes and subcortical regions, thus supporting the theory that neurodegeneration might be driven by a selective vulnerability of large-scale brain functional networks [155].

In nfvPPA, selective functional changes within the left fronto-insular speech production network (SPN, involving the frontal operculum, primary and supplementary motor areas and inferior parietal lobule) have been shown to precede structural alterations [156]. Focal neurodegeneration within the SPN in nfvPPA has been recently associated with network-specific topological functional alterations, providing evidence of a network-based degeneration also in this clinical syndrome [155]. In svPPA, reduced functional connectivity was shown to particularly affect a semantic network centered on the left anterior temporal lobe and also involving widespread interconnected modality-selective regions in the sensory, motor, and association cortices [157]. Network-based analysis has also shown that the focal degeneration of anterior temporal and perisylvian regions in svPPA is accompanied by a distributed pattern of functional network topological alterations in inferior and ventral regions of the temporal lobe, bilateral frontal cortex, left amygdala, hippocampus, caudate, and occipital regions [158].

In summary, although RS fMRI has proven robust in differentiating bvFTD from AD [149], more research is needed to allow for a large-scale application of this technique at a single-subject level in all the clinical variants of the FTLD spectrum.

3.2.4 Neuroimaging in Presymptomatic FTLD

Approximately 30% of FTLD cases are familial, usually associated with mutations in a handful of genes [159], suggesting that therapeutic intervention targeted against each genetic alteration might be useful, particularly in the presymptomatic phases. Therefore, validating imaging biomarkers of early structural and functional alterations in genetically determined FTLD is essential for the design of future pharmacological trials targeting these conditions.

The entity of gray matter atrophy in presymptomatic FTLD-related mutation carriers is debated, as some early single-case reports showed mild atrophy in the different mutation types [160–162], whereas more recent studies performed in sizeable cohorts suggested a more complex evolution of structural alterations over time according to the underlying mutation, with *MAPT* or *GRN* mutation carriers not showing significant structural abnormalities before the symptom onset [152, 163–165], and presymptomatic *C9orf72* repeat expansion carriers demonstrating some gray matter atrophy in the cerebellum and insula [165]. A major limitation that probably contributes to inconsistencies across these studies is the small sample size. The Genetic Frontotemporal Dementia Initiative (GENFI) international consortium has recently tried to overcome such limitation, demonstrating significant differences in cortical and subcortical volumes between presymptomatic carriers and non-carriers that occurred more than 10 years before expected clinical onset, with the earliest changes observed in the insula, closely followed by the temporal and then frontal lobes [166].

Some recent studies have suggested that other imaging techniques assessing structural and functional connectivity may detect earlier alterations than atrophy, and therefore show greater utility as early markers. DT MRI has shown diffuse degeneration of frontal and temporal tracts in presymptomatic carriers of *GRN* [167, 168], *MAPT* [164, 168], and *C9orf72* mutations [168, 169], with a distinctive damage to the posterior thalamic radiations [168] and corticospinal tracts [169] when the *C9orf72* expansion was present. A recent study of the GENFI consortium showed that diffusion changes in *C9orf72* mutation carriers are present significantly earlier than both *MAPT* and *GRN* mutation carriers, up to 30 years before the estimated onset of symptoms [168].

Functional techniques such as FDG-PET and fMRI have demonstrated significant abnormalities in the presymptomatic stages of FTLD. In fact, asymmetrical hypometabolism was found in the frontal and temporal lobes of asymptomatic *GRN* carriers before the onset of clinical symptoms and gray matter atrophy [103, 104]. Using RS fMRI, presymptomatic *MAPT* mutation carriers showed no abnormalities of the salience network, whereas the DMN displayed a reduced connectivity of lateral temporal and medial prefrontal nodes and an increased connectivity of other components of the network (medial parietal) [152]. On the contrary, presymptomatic *GRN* mutation carriers showed an increased connectivity of the salience network, with no abnormalities of the DMN [163]. A larger RS fMRI study showed a reduced functional connectivity of the anterior mid-cingulate cortex in both *MAPT* and *GRN* mutation carriers with no alterations of the posterior cingulate connectivity [164]. So far, only one study has assessed functional connectivity in presymptomatic *C9orf72* expansion carriers, demonstrating prominent connectivity disruption in the salience and medial pulvinar thalamus-seeded networks [169]. Despite some inconsistencies, all these studies showed absent or minimal gray matter atrophy [152, 163, 164, 169], suggesting that RS fMRI changes may predate atrophy.

3.3   Clinical Case #1

A 69-year-old man was conducted to medical attention by his family members, as he was almost completely acritical toward his own cognitive difficulties. Caregivers reported a 4-year history of attention and memory problems with a rapid worsening over time. Mood swings, diminished social interest, and loss of empathy were

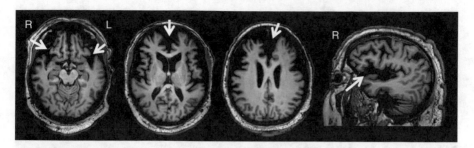

Fig. 3.9   T1-weighted MR images from clinical case #1 showing sulcal enlargement (arrows) due to severe, bilateral atrophy of the frontal lobes. *L* left, *R* right

reported. In the last 2 years, the patient also showed frequent gnashing of teeth, increased dietary intake, and a significant increase in the number of cigarettes he smokes per day. Neuropsychological testing showed severe, multidomain cognitive impairment with relative sparing of visuospatial abilities. MRI scan displayed a severe, bilateral atrophy of frontal lobes (Fig. 3.9). Cerebrospinal fluid (CSF) analysis was negative for biomarkers of AD pathology. This patient received a diagnosis of probable bvFTD [2].

3.4   Clinical Case #2

A 67-year-old man presented with a 4-year history of progressive cognitive difficulties mainly regarding short-term memory and concentration. Family members also reported significant behavioral disturbances that accompanied the appearance of cognitive symptoms, including disinhibition, irritability, and emotional lability. He also showed worsening apathy and indifference toward his previous interests and close friends. Dietary changes and stereotypy of speech were also reported. Neuropsychological testing performed at clinical presentation showed a multidomain cognitive impairment, with prominent involvement of executive functions and sustained attention and milder memory deficits, although global cognitive functioning measured using the Mini Mental State Examination (MMSE) was within the normal range (27/30). MRI scan showed mild atrophy of bilateral anterior temporal, perisylvian, and dorsolateral frontal cortical structures, with a slight prevalence in the left hemisphere (Fig. 3.10a). FDG-PET showed moderate hypometabolism in the anterior temporal structures and sparing of posterior cortical structures (Fig. 3.10b). The patient denied consent to CSF sampling and analysis. Therefore, amyloid PET with ^{11}C-PiB was performed, showing severe amyloid deposition in the brain (Fig. 3.10c). Considering the presence of a biomarker strongly indicative of AD pathology in a patient with early-onset cognitive and behavioral syndrome, he was diagnosed with a frontal presentation of AD.

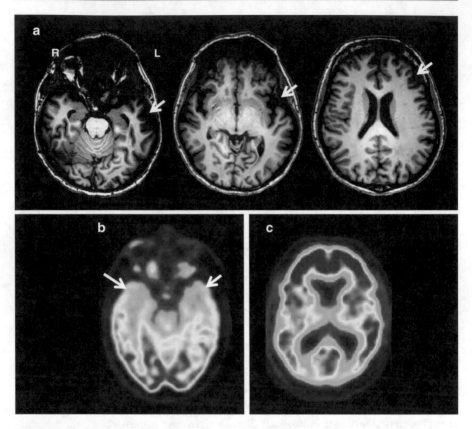

Fig. 3.10 T1-weighted MR images from clinical case #2 showing mild atrophy of bilateral anterior temporal, perisylvian, and dorsolateral frontal cortex, with a left hemispheric prevalence (**a**, arrows). FDG-PET scan demonstrating bilateral anterior temporal hypometabolism (**b**, arrows). Amyloid PET scan showing severe amyloid deposition (**c**). *L* left, *R* right

References

1. Neary D, Snowden JS, Gustafson L, et al. Frontotemporal lobar degeneration: a consensus on clinical diagnostic criteria. Neurology. 1998;51:1546–54.
2. Rascovsky K, Hodges JR, Knopman D, et al. Sensitivity of revised diagnostic criteria for the behavioural variant of frontotemporal dementia. Brain. 2011;134:2456–77.
3. Josephs KA, Duffy JR, Strand EA, et al. Clinicopathological and imaging correlates of progressive aphasia and apraxia of speech. Brain. 2006;129:1385–98.
4. Gorno-Tempini ML, Hillis AE, Weintraub S, et al. Classification of primary progressive aphasia and its variants. Neurology. 2011;76:1006–14.
5. Gorno-Tempini ML, Dronkers NF, Rankin KP, et al. Cognition and anatomy in three variants of primary progressive aphasia. Ann Neurol. 2004;55:335–46.
6. Rohrer JD, Warren JD, Modat M, et al. Patterns of cortical thinning in the language variants of frontotemporal lobar degeneration. Neurology. 2009;72:1562–9.
7. Hodges JR, Patterson K. Semantic dementia: a unique clinicopathological syndrome. Lancet Neurol. 2007;6:1004–14.

8. Seelaar H, Rohrer JD, Pijnenburg YA, Fox NC, van Swieten JC. Clinical, genetic and pathological heterogeneity of frontotemporal dementia: a review. J Neurol Neurosurg Psychiatry. 2011;82:476–86.
9. Wilhelmsen KC. Frontotemporal dementia is on the MAPtau. Ann Neurol. 1997;41:139–40.
10. Hutton M, Lewis J, Dickson D, Yen SH, McGowan E. Analysis of tauopathies with transgenic mice. Trends Mol Med. 2001;7:467–70.
11. Neumann M, Sampathu DM, Kwong LK, et al. Ubiquitinated TDP-43 in frontotemporal lobar degeneration and amyotrophic lateral sclerosis. Science. 2006;314:130–3.
12. Baker M, Mackenzie IR, Pickering-Brown SM, et al. Mutations in progranulin cause tau-negative frontotemporal dementia linked to chromosome 17. Nature. 2006;442:916–9.
13. Rohrer JD, Isaacs AM, Mizielinska S, et al. *C9orf72* expansions in frontotemporal dementia and amyotrophic lateral sclerosis. Lancet Neurol. 2015;14:291–301.
14. Neumann M, Rademakers R, Roeber S, et al. A new subtype of frontotemporal lobar degeneration with FUS pathology. Brain. 2009;132:2922–31.
15. Rosen HJ, Gorno-Tempini ML, Goldman WP, et al. Patterns of brain atrophy in frontotemporal dementia and semantic dementia. Neurology. 2002;58:198–208.
16. Boccardi M, Sabattoli F, Laakso MP, et al. Frontotemporal dementia as a neural system disease. Neurobiol Aging. 2005;26:37–44.
17. Perry RJ, Graham A, Williams G, et al. Patterns of frontal lobe atrophy in frontotemporal dementia: a volumetric MRI study. Dement Geriatr Cogn Disord. 2006;22:278–87.
18. Du AT, Schuff N, Kramer JH, et al. Different regional patterns of cortical thinning in Alzheimer's disease and frontotemporal dementia. Brain. 2007;130:1159–66.
19. Seeley WW, Crawford R, Rascovsky K, et al. Frontal paralimbic network atrophy in very mild behavioral variant frontotemporal dementia. Arch Neurol. 2008;65:249–55.
20. Rabinovici GD, Seeley WW, Kim EJ, et al. Distinct MRI atrophy patterns in autopsy-proven Alzheimer's disease and frontotemporal lobar degeneration. Am J Alzheimers Dis Other Dement. 2007;22:474–88.
21. Borroni B, Brambati SM, Agosti C, et al. Evidence of white matter changes on diffusion tensor imaging in frontotemporal dementia. Arch Neurol. 2007;64:246–51.
22. Cardenas VA, Boxer AL, Chao LL, et al. Deformation-based morphometry reveals brain atrophy in frontotemporal dementia. Arch Neurol. 2007;64:873–7.
23. Chao LL, Schuff N, Clevenger EM, et al. Patterns of white matter atrophy in frontotemporal lobar degeneration. Arch Neurol. 2007;64:1619–24.
24. Schroeter ML, Raczka K, Neumann J, Yves von Cramon D. Towards a nosology for frontotemporal lobar degenerations-a meta-analysis involving 267 subjects. NeuroImage. 2007;36:497–510.
25. Harris JM, Gall C, Thompson JC, et al. Sensitivity and specificity of FTDC criteria for behavioral variant frontotemporal dementia. Neurology. 2013;80:1881–7.
26. Schroeter ML, Laird AR, Chwiesko C, et al. Conceptualizing neuropsychiatric diseases with multimodal data-driven meta-analyses—the case of behavioral variant frontotemporal dementia. Cortex. 2014;57:22–37.
27. Whitwell JL, Przybelski SA, Weigand SD, et al. Distinct anatomical subtypes of the behavioural variant of frontotemporal dementia: a cluster analysis study. Brain. 2009;132:2932–46.
28. Shimizu H, Hokoishi K, Fukuhara R, Komori K, Ikeda M. Two cases of frontotemporal dementia with predominant temporal lobe atrophy. Psychogeriatrics. 2009;9:204–7.
29. Murray ME, Kouri N, Lin WL, et al. Clinicopathologic assessment and imaging of tauopathies in neurodegenerative dementias. Alzheimers Res Ther. 2014;6:1.
30. Rankin KP, Mayo MC, Seeley WW, et al. Behavioral variant frontotemporal dementia with corticobasal degeneration pathology: phenotypic comparison to bvFTD with Pick's disease. J Mol Neurosci. 2011;45:594–608.
31. Josephs KA, Whitwell JL, Dickson DW, et al. Voxel-based morphometry in autopsy proven PSP and CBD. Neurobiol Aging. 2008;29:280–9.

32. Boxer AL, Geschwind MD, Belfor N, et al. Patterns of brain atrophy that differentiate corticobasal degeneration syndrome from progressive supranuclear palsy. Arch Neurol. 2006;63:81–6.
33. Whitwell JL, Jack CR Jr, Boeve BF, et al. Voxel-based morphometry patterns of atrophy in FTLD with mutations in MAPT or PGRN. Neurology. 2009;72:813–20.
34. Rohrer JD, Ridgway GR, Modat M, et al. Distinct profiles of brain atrophy in frontotemporal lobar degeneration caused by progranulin and tau mutations. NeuroImage. 2010;53:1070–6.
35. Perry DC, Brown JA, Possin KL, et al. Clinicopathological correlations in behavioural variant frontotemporal dementia. Brain. 2017;140:3329–45.
36. Bocchetta M, Cardoso MJ, Cash DM, et al. Patterns of regional cerebellar atrophy in genetic frontotemporal dementia. Neuroimage Clin. 2016;11:287–90.
37. Whitwell JL, Boeve BF, Weigand SD, et al. Brain atrophy over time in genetic and sporadic frontotemporal dementia: a study of 198 serial magnetic resonance images. Eur J Neurol. 2015;22:745–52.
38. Rohrer JD, Rosen HJ. Neuroimaging in frontotemporal dementia. Int Rev Psychiatry. 2013;25:221–9.
39. Murray ME, DeJesus-Hernandez M, Rutherford NJ, et al. Clinical and neuropathologic heterogeneity of c9FTD/ALS associated with hexanucleotide repeat expansion in *C9ORF72*. Acta Neuropathol. 2011;122:673–90.
40. Snowden JS, Rollinson S, Thompson JC, et al. Distinct clinical and pathological characteristics of frontotemporal dementia associated with *C9ORF72* mutations. Brain. 2012;135:693–708.
41. Mackenzie IR, Neumann M. Subcortical TDP-43 pathology patterns validate cortical FTLD-TDP subtypes and demonstrate unique aspects of *C9orf72* mutation cases. Acta Neuropathol. 2020;139:83–98.
42. Mahoney CJ, Beck J, Rohrer JD, et al. Frontotemporal dementia with the *C9ORF72* hexanucleotide repeat expansion: clinical, neuroanatomical and neuropathological features. Brain. 2012;135:736–50.
43. Whitwell JL, Weigand SD, Boeve BF, et al. Neuroimaging signatures of frontotemporal dementia genetics: *C9ORF72*, tau, progranulin and sporadics. Brain. 2012;135:794–806.
44. Boxer AL, Mackenzie IR, Boeve BF, et al. Clinical, neuroimaging and neuropathological features of a new chromosome 9p-linked FTD-ALS family. J Neurol Neurosurg Psychiatry. 2011;82:196–203.
45. Agosta F, Ferraro PM, Riva N, et al. Structural and functional brain signatures of *C9orf72* in motor neuron disease. Neurobiol Aging. 2017;57:206–19.
46. Bede P, Omer T, Finegan E, et al. Connectivity-based characterisation of subcortical grey matter pathology in frontotemporal dementia and ALS: a multimodal neuroimaging study. Brain Imaging Behav. 2018;12:1696–707.
47. Bocchetta M, Iglesias JE, Neason M, et al. Thalamic nuclei in frontotemporal dementia: Mediodorsal nucleus involvement is universal but pulvinar atrophy is unique to *C9orf72*. Hum Brain Mapp. 2020;41:1006–16.
48. Karageorgiou E, Miller BL. Frontotemporal lobar degeneration: a clinical approach. Semin Neurol. 2014;34:189–201.
49. Lee SE, Seeley WW, Poorzand P, et al. Clinical characterization of bvFTD due to FUS neuropathology. Neurocase. 2012;18:305–17.
50. Josephs KA, Whitwell JL, Parisi JE, et al. Caudate atrophy on MRI is a characteristic feature of FTLD-FUS. Eur J Neurol. 2010;17:969–75.
51. Snowden JS, Hu Q, Rollinson S, et al. The most common type of FTLD-FUS (aFTLD-U) is associated with a distinct clinical form of frontotemporal dementia but is not related to mutations in the FUS gene. Acta Neuropathol. 2011;122:99–110.
52. Agosta F, Canu E, Sarro L, Comi G, Filippi M. Neuroimaging findings in frontotemporal lobar degeneration spectrum of disorders. Cortex. 2012;48:389–413.
53. Varma AR, Adams W, Lloyd JJ, et al. Diagnostic patterns of regional atrophy on MRI and regional cerebral blood flow change on SPECT in young onset patients with Alzheimer's disease, frontotemporal dementia and vascular dementia. Acta Neurol Scand. 2002;105:261–9.

54. Likeman M, Anderson VM, Stevens JM, et al. Visual assessment of atrophy on magnetic resonance imaging in the diagnosis of pathologically confirmed young-onset dementias. Arch Neurol. 2005;62:1410–5.
55. Lehmann M, Rohrer JD, Clarkson MJ, et al. Reduced cortical thickness in the posterior cingulate gyrus is characteristic of both typical and atypical Alzheimer's disease. J Alzheimers Dis. 2010;20:587–98.
56. Whitwell JL, Jack CR Jr, Przybelski SA, et al. Temporoparietal atrophy: a marker of AD pathology independent of clinical diagnosis. Neurobiol Aging. 2011;32:1531–41.
57. Canu E, Agosta F, Mandic-Stojmenovic G, et al. Multiparametric MRI to distinguish early onset Alzheimer's disease and behavioural variant of frontotemporal dementia. Neuroimage Clin. 2017;15:428–38.
58. Davies RR, Kipps CM, Mitchell J, et al. Progression in frontotemporal dementia: identifying a benign behavioral variant by magnetic resonance imaging. Arch Neurol. 2006;63:1627–31.
59. Kipps CM, Davies RR, Mitchell J, et al. Clinical significance of lobar atrophy in frontotemporal dementia: application of an MRI visual rating scale. Dement Geriatr Cogn Disord. 2007;23:334–42.
60. Josephs KA, Whitwell JL, Jack CR, Parisi JE, Dickson DW. Frontotemporal lobar degeneration without lobar atrophy. Arch Neurol. 2006;63:1632–8.
61. Rogalski E, Cobia D, Harrison TM, et al. Progression of language decline and cortical atrophy in subtypes of primary progressive aphasia. Neurology. 2011;76:1804–10.
62. Garibotto V, Borroni B, Agosti C, et al. Subcortical and deep cortical atrophy in frontotemporal lobar degeneration. Neurobiol Aging. 2011;32:875–84.
63. van de Pol LA, Hensel A, van der Flier WM, et al. Hippocampal atrophy on MRI in frontotemporal lobar degeneration and Alzheimer's disease. J Neurol Neurosurg Psychiatry. 2006;77:439–42.
64. Mummery CJ, Patterson K, Price CJ, et al. A voxel-based morphometry study of semantic dementia: relationship between temporal lobe atrophy and semantic memory. Ann Neurol. 2000;47:36–45.
65. Galton CJ, Patterson K, Graham K, et al. Differing patterns of temporal atrophy in Alzheimer's disease and semantic dementia. Neurology. 2001;57:216–25.
66. Chan D, Fox NC, Scahill RI, et al. Patterns of temporal lobe atrophy in semantic dementia and Alzheimer's disease. Ann Neurol. 2001;49:433–42.
67. Boxer AL, Miller BL. Clinical features of frontotemporal dementia. Alzheimer Dis Assoc Disord. 2005;19(Suppl 1):S3–6.
68. Collins JA, Montal V, Hochberg D, et al. Focal temporal pole atrophy and network degeneration in semantic variant primary progressive aphasia. Brain. 2017;140:457–71.
69. Josephs KA, Whitwell JL, Knopman DS, et al. Two distinct subtypes of right temporal variant frontotemporal dementia. Neurology. 2009;73:1443–50.
70. Brambati SM, Rankin KP, Narvid J, et al. Atrophy progression in semantic dementia with asymmetric temporal involvement: a tensor-based morphometry study. Neurobiol Aging. 2009;30:103–11.
71. Chare L, Hodges JR, Leyton CE, et al. New criteria for frontotemporal dementia syndromes: clinical and pathological diagnostic implications. J Neurol Neurosurg Psychiatry. 2014;85:865–70.
72. Grossman M. Primary progressive aphasia: clinicopathological correlations. Nat Rev Neurol. 2010;6:88–97.
73. Spinelli EG, Mandelli ML, Miller ZA, et al. Typical and atypical pathology in primary progressive aphasia variants. Ann Neurol. 2017;81:430–43.
74. Rohrer JD, Lashley T, Schott JM, et al. Clinical and neuroanatomical signatures of tissue pathology in frontotemporal lobar degeneration. Brain. 2011;134:2565–81.
75. Hodges JR, Mitchell J, Dawson K, et al. Semantic dementia: demography, familial factors and survival in a consecutive series of 100 cases. Brain. 2010;133:300–6.
76. Mesulam M, Wicklund A, Johnson N, et al. Alzheimer and frontotemporal pathology in subsets of primary progressive aphasia. Ann Neurol. 2008;63:709–19.

77. Josephs KA, Whitwell JL, Duffy JR, et al. Progressive aphasia secondary to Alzheimer disease vs FTLD pathology. Neurology. 2008;70:25–34.
78. Canu E, Agosta F, Imperiale F, et al. Added value of multimodal MRI to the clinical diagnosis of primary progressive aphasia variants. Cortex. 2019;113:58–66.
79. Rohrer JD, Rossor MN, Warren JD. Alzheimer's pathology in primary progressive aphasia. Neurobiol Aging. 2012;33:744–52.
80. Agosta F, Ferraro PM, Canu E, et al. Differentiation between subtypes of primary progressive aphasia by using cortical thickness and diffusion-tensor MR imaging measures. Radiology. 2015;276:219–27.
81. Jeong Y, Cho SS, Park JM, et al. 18F-FDG PET findings in frontotemporal dementia: an SPM analysis of 29 patients. J Nucl Med. 2005;46:233–9.
82. Grimmer T, Diehl J, Drzezga A, Forstl H, Kurz A. Region-specific decline of cerebral glucose metabolism in patients with frontotemporal dementia: a prospective 18F-FDG-PET study. Dement Geriatr Cogn Disord. 2004;18:32–6.
83. Ishii K, Sakamoto S, Sasaki M, et al. Cerebral glucose metabolism in patients with frontotemporal dementia. J Nucl Med. 1998;39:1875–8.
84. Mendez MF, Shapira JS, McMurtray A, Licht E, Miller BL. Accuracy of the clinical evaluation for frontotemporal dementia. Arch Neurol. 2007;64:830–5.
85. Morbelli S, Ferrara M, Fiz F, et al. Mapping brain morphological and functional conversion patterns in predementia late-onset bvFTD. Eur J Nucl Med Mol Imaging. 2016;43:1337–47.
86. Diehl-Schmid J, Grimmer T, Drzezga A, et al. Decline of cerebral glucose metabolism in frontotemporal dementia: a longitudinal 18F-FDG-PET-study. Neurobiol Aging. 2007;28:42–50.
87. Sjogren M, Gustafson L, Wikkelso C, Wallin A. Frontotemporal dementia can be distinguished from Alzheimer's disease and subcortical white matter dementia by an anterior-to-posterior rCBF-SPET ratio. Dement Geriatr Cogn Disord. 2000;11:275–85.
88. Ibach B, Poljansky S, Marienhagen J, et al. Contrasting metabolic impairment in frontotemporal degeneration and early onset Alzheimer's disease. NeuroImage. 2004;23:739–43.
89. Charpentier P, Lavenu I, Defebvre L, et al. Alzheimer's disease and frontotemporal dementia are differentiated by discriminant analysis applied to (99m)Tc HmPAO SPECT data. J Neurol Neurosurg Psychiatry. 2000;69:661–3.
90. Kanda T, Ishii K, Uemura T, et al. Comparison of grey matter and metabolic reductions in frontotemporal dementia using FDG-PET and voxel-based morphometric MR studies. Eur J Nucl Med Mol Imaging. 2008;35:2227–34.
91. McNeill R, Sare GM, Manoharan M, et al. Accuracy of single-photon emission computed tomography in differentiating frontotemporal dementia from Alzheimer's disease. J Neurol Neurosurg Psychiatry. 2007;78:350–5.
92. Womack KB, Diaz-Arrastia R, Aizenstein HJ, et al. Temporoparietal hypometabolism in frontotemporal lobar degeneration and associated imaging diagnostic errors. Arch Neurol. 2011;68:329–37.
93. Tosun D, Schuff N, Rabinovici GD, et al. Diagnostic utility of ASL-MRI and FDG-PET in the behavioral variant of FTD and AD. Ann Clin Transl Neurol. 2016;3:740–51.
94. Vijverberg EG, Wattjes MP, Dols A, et al. Diagnostic accuracy of MRI and additional [18F]FDG-PET for behavioral variant frontotemporal dementia in patients with late onset behavioral changes. J Alzheimers Dis. 2016;53:1287–97.
95. Buhour MS, Doidy F, Laisney M, et al. Pathophysiology of the behavioral variant of frontotemporal lobar degeneration: a study combining MRI and FDG-PET. Brain Imaging Behav. 2017;11:240–52.
96. Rabinovici GD, Jagust WJ, Furst AJ, et al. Abeta amyloid and glucose metabolism in three variants of primary progressive aphasia. Ann Neurol. 2008;64:388–401.
97. Nestor PJ, Graham NL, Fryer TD, et al. Progressive non-fluent aphasia is associated with hypometabolism centred on the left anterior insula. Brain. 2003;126:2406–18.
98. Zahn R, Buechert M, Overmans J, et al. Mapping of temporal and parietal cortex in progressive nonfluent aphasia and Alzheimer's disease using chemical shift imaging, voxel-based morphometry and positron emission tomography. Psychiatry Res. 2005;140:115–31.

99. Perneczky R, Diehl-Schmid J, Pohl C, Drzezga A, Kurz A. Non-fluent progressive aphasia: cerebral metabolic patterns and brain reserve. Brain Res. 2007;1133:178–85.
100. Nestor PJ, Balan K, Cheow HK, et al. Nuclear imaging can predict pathologic diagnosis in progressive nonfluent aphasia. Neurology. 2007;68:238–9.
101. Nestor PJ, Fryer TD, Hodges JR. Declarative memory impairments in Alzheimer's disease and semantic dementia. NeuroImage. 2006;30:1010–20.
102. Drzezga A, Grimmer T, Henriksen G, et al. Imaging of amyloid plaques and cerebral glucose metabolism in semantic dementia and Alzheimer's disease. NeuroImage. 2008;39:619–33.
103. Jacova C, Hsiung GY, Tawankanjanachot I, et al. Anterior brain glucose hypometabolism predates dementia in progranulin mutation carriers. Neurology. 2013;81:1322–31.
104. Caroppo P, Habert MO, Durrleman S, et al. Lateral temporal lobe: an early imaging marker of the presymptomatic GRN disease? J Alzheimers Dis. 2015;47:751–9.
105. Cistaro A, Pagani M, Montuschi A, et al. The metabolic signature of C9ORF72-related ALS: FDG PET comparison with nonmutated patients. Eur J Nucl Med Mol Imaging. 2014;41:844–52.
106. Deters KD, Risacher SL, Farlow MR, et al. Cerebral hypometabolism and grey matter density in MAPT intron 10 +3 mutation carriers. Am J Neurodegener Dis. 2014;3:103–14.
107. Chételat G, Arbizu J, Barthel H, et al. Amyloid-PET and ^{18}F-FDG-PET in the diagnostic investigation of Alzheimer's disease and other dementias. Lancet Neurol. 2020;19:951–62.
108. Rowe CC, Ng S, Ackermann U, et al. Imaging beta-amyloid burden in aging and dementia. Neurology. 2007;68:1718–25.
109. Rabinovici GD, Furst AJ, O'Neil JP, et al. 11C-PIB PET imaging in Alzheimer disease and frontotemporal lobar degeneration. Neurology. 2007;68:1205–12.
110. Engler H, Santillo AF, Wang SX, et al. In vivo amyloid imaging with PET in frontotemporal dementia. Eur J Nucl Med Mol Imaging. 2008;35:100–6.
111. Leyton CE, Villemagne VL, Savage S, et al. Subtypes of progressive aphasia: application of the International Consensus Criteria and validation using beta-amyloid imaging. Brain. 2011;134:3030–43.
112. Rabinovici GD, Rosen HJ, Alkalay A, et al. Amyloid vs FDG-PET in the differential diagnosis of AD and FTLD. Neurology. 2011;77:2034–42.
113. Rowe CC, Ackerman U, Browne W, et al. Imaging of amyloid beta in Alzheimer's disease with 18F-BAY94-9172, a novel PET tracer: proof of mechanism. Lancet Neurol. 2008;7:129–35.
114. Villemagne VL, Ong K, Mulligan RS, et al. Amyloid imaging with (18)F-florbetaben in Alzheimer disease and other dementias. J Nucl Med. 2011;52:1210–7.
115. Mesulam MM, Weintraub S, Rogalski EJ, et al. Asymmetry and heterogeneity of Alzheimer's and frontotemporal pathology in primary progressive aphasia. Brain. 2014;137:1176–92.
116. Bergeron D, Gorno-Tempini ML, Rabinovici GD, et al. Prevalence of amyloid-beta pathology in distinct variants of primary progressive aphasia. Ann Neurol. 2018;84:729–40.
117. Ossenkoppele R, Jansen WJ, Rabinovici GD, et al. Prevalence of amyloid PET positivity in dementia syndromes: a meta-analysis. JAMA. 2015;313:1939–49.
118. Jansen WJ, Ossenkoppele R, Knol DL, et al. Prevalence of cerebral amyloid pathology in persons without dementia: a meta-analysis. JAMA. 2015;313:1924–38.
119. Leuzy A, Chiotis K, Lemoine L, et al. Tau PET imaging in neurodegenerative tauopathies-still a challenge. Mol Psychiatry. 2019;24:1112–34.
120. Kikuchi A, Okamura N, Hasegawa T, et al. In vivo visualization of tau deposits in corticobasal syndrome by 18F-THK5351 PET. Neurology. 2016;87:2309–16.
121. Smith R, Scholl M, Widner H, et al. In vivo retention of (18)F-AV-1451 in corticobasal syndrome. Neurology. 2017;89:845–53.
122. Whitwell JL, Lowe VJ, Tosakulwong N, et al. [(18) F]AV-1451 tau positron emission tomography in progressive supranuclear palsy. Mov Disord. 2017;32:124–33.
123. Schonhaut DR, McMillan CT, Spina S, et al. (18) F-flortaucipir tau positron emission tomography distinguishes established progressive supranuclear palsy from controls and Parkinson disease: a multicenter study. Ann Neurol. 2017;82:622–34.

124. Passamonti L, Vazquez Rodriguez P, Hong YT, et al. 18F-AV-1451 positron emission tomography in Alzheimer's disease and progressive supranuclear palsy. Brain. 2017;140:781–91.
125. Smith R, Schain M, Nilsson C, et al. Increased basal ganglia binding of (18) F-AV-1451 in patients with progressive supranuclear palsy. Mov Disord. 2017;32:108–14.
126. Bevan-Jones WR, Cope TE, Jones PS, et al. [(18)F]AV-1451 binding in vivo mirrors the expected distribution of TDP-43 pathology in the semantic variant of primary progressive aphasia. J Neurol Neurosurg Psychiatry. 2018;89:1032–7.
127. Josephs KA, Martin PR, Botha H, et al. [(18) F]AV-1451 tau-PET and primary progressive aphasia. Ann Neurol. 2018;83:599–611.
128. Neumann M, Kwong LK, Truax AC, et al. TDP-43-positive white matter pathology in frontotemporal lobar degeneration with ubiquitin-positive inclusions. J Neuropathol Exp Neurol. 2007;66:177–83.
129. Mackenzie IR, Neumann M. Molecular neuropathology of frontotemporal dementia: insights into disease mechanisms from postmortem studies. J Neurochem. 2016;138(Suppl 1):54–70.
130. Caroppo P, Le Ber I, Camuzat A, et al. Extensive white matter involvement in patients with frontotemporal lobar degeneration: think progranulin. JAMA Neurol. 2014;71:1562–6.
131. Sudre CH, Bocchetta M, Cash D, et al. White matter hyperintensities are seen only in GRN mutation carriers in the GENFI cohort. Neuroimage Clin. 2017;15:171–80.
132. Woollacott IOC, Bocchetta M, Sudre CH, et al. Pathological correlates of white matter hyperintensities in a case of progranulin mutation associated frontotemporal dementia. Neurocase. 2018;24:166–74.
133. Agosta F, Scola E, Canu E, et al. White matter damage in frontotemporal lobar degeneration spectrum. Cereb Cortex. 2012;22:2705–14.
134. Whitwell JL, Avula R, Senjem ML, et al. Gray and white matter water diffusion in the syndromic variants of frontotemporal dementia. Neurology. 2010;74:1279–87.
135. Zhang Y, Schuff N, Du AT, et al. White matter damage in frontotemporal dementia and Alzheimer's disease measured by diffusion MRI. Brain. 2009;132:2579–92.
136. Zhang Y, Tartaglia MC, Schuff N, et al. MRI signatures of brain macrostructural atrophy and microstructural degradation in frontotemporal lobar degeneration subtypes. J Alzheimers Dis. 2013;33:431–44.
137. Mahoney CJ, Ridgway GR, Malone IB, et al. Profiles of white matter tract pathology in frontotemporal dementia. Hum Brain Mapp. 2014;35:4163–79.
138. McMillan CT, Irwin DJ, Avants BB, et al. White matter imaging helps dissociate tau from TDP-43 in frontotemporal lobar degeneration. J Neurol Neurosurg Psychiatry. 2013;84:949–55.
139. Agosta F, Galantucci S, Magnani G, et al. MRI signatures of the frontotemporal lobar degeneration continuum. Hum Brain Mapp. 2015;36:2602–14.
140. Avants BB, Cook PA, Ungar L, Gee JC, Grossman M. Dementia induces correlated reductions in white matter integrity and cortical thickness: a multivariate neuroimaging study with sparse canonical correlation analysis. NeuroImage. 2010;50:1004–16.
141. Galantucci S, Tartaglia MC, Wilson SM, et al. White matter damage in primary progressive aphasias: a diffusion tensor tractography study. Brain. 2011;134:3011–29.
142. Schwindt GC, Graham NL, Rochon E, et al. Whole-brain white matter disruption in semantic and nonfluent variants of primary progressive aphasia. Hum Brain Mapp. 2013;34:973–84.
143. Mahoney CJ, Malone IB, Ridgway GR, et al. White matter tract signatures of the progressive aphasias. Neurobiol Aging. 2013;34:1687–99.
144. Mandelli ML, Caverzasi E, Binney RJ, et al. Frontal white matter tracts sustaining speech production in primary progressive aphasia. J Neurosci. 2014;34:9754–67.
145. Catani M, Mesulam MM, Jakobsen E, et al. A novel frontal pathway underlies verbal fluency in primary progressive aphasia. Brain. 2013;136:2619–28.
146. Acosta-Cabronero J, Patterson K, Fryer TD, et al. Atrophy, hypometabolism and white matter abnormalities in semantic dementia tell a coherent story. Brain. 2011;134:2025–35.
147. Agosta F, Galantucci S, Canu E, et al. Disruption of structural connectivity along the dorsal and ventral language pathways in patients with nonfluent and semantic variant primary progressive aphasia: a DT MRI study and a literature review. Brain Lang. 2013;127:157–66.

148. Agosta F, Henry RG, Migliaccio R, et al. Language networks in semantic dementia. Brain. 2010;133:286–99.
149. Zhou J, Greicius MD, Gennatas ED, et al. Divergent network connectivity changes in behavioural variant frontotemporal dementia and Alzheimer's disease. Brain. 2010;133:1352–67.
150. Farb NA, Grady CL, Strother S, et al. Abnormal network connectivity in frontotemporal dementia: evidence for prefrontal isolation. Cortex. 2013;49:1856–73.
151. Filippi M, Agosta F, Scola E, et al. Functional network connectivity in the behavioral variant of frontotemporal dementia. Cortex. 2013;49:2389–401.
152. Whitwell JL, Josephs KA, Avula R, et al. Altered functional connectivity in asymptomatic MAPT subjects: a comparison to bvFTD. Neurology. 2011;77:866–74.
153. Seeley WW, Menon V, Schatzberg AF, et al. Dissociable intrinsic connectivity networks for salience processing and executive control. J Neurosci. 2007;27:2349–56.
154. Agosta F, Sala S, Valsasina P, et al. Brain network connectivity assessed using graph theory in frontotemporal dementia. Neurology. 2013;81:134–43.
155. Seeley WW, Crawford RK, Zhou J, Miller BL, Greicius MD. Neurodegenerative diseases target large-scale human brain networks. Neuron. 2009;62:42–52.
156. Bonakdarpour B, Rogalski EJ, Wang A, et al. Functional connectivity is reduced in early-stage primary progressive aphasia when atrophy is not prominent. Alzheimer Dis Assoc Disord. 2017;31:101–6.
157. Guo CC, Gorno-Tempini ML, Gesierich B, et al. Anterior temporal lobe degeneration produces widespread network-driven dysfunction. Brain. 2013;136:2979–91.
158. Agosta F, Galantucci S, Valsasina P, et al. Disrupted brain connectome in semantic variant of primary progressive aphasia. Neurobiol Aging. 2014;35:2646–55.
159. Ferrari R, Manzoni C, Hardy J. Genetics and molecular mechanisms of frontotemporal lobar degeneration: an update and future avenues. Neurobiol Aging. 2019;78:98–110.
160. Janssen JC, Schott JM, Cipolotti L, et al. Mapping the onset and progression of atrophy in familial frontotemporal lobar degeneration. J Neurol Neurosurg Psychiatry. 2005;76:162–8.
161. Rohrer JD, Warren JD, Barnes J, et al. Mapping the progression of progranulin-associated frontotemporal lobar degeneration. Nat Clin Pract Neurol. 2008;4:455–60.
162. Spina S, Farlow MR, Unverzagt FW, et al. The tauopathy associated with mutation +3 in intron 10 of tau: characterization of the MSTD family. Brain. 2008;131:72–89.
163. Borroni B, Alberici A, Cercignani M, et al. Granulin mutation drives brain damage and reorganization from preclinical to symptomatic FTLD. Neurobiol Aging. 2012;33:2506–20.
164. Dopper EG, Rombouts SA, Jiskoot LC, et al. Structural and functional brain connectivity in presymptomatic familial frontotemporal dementia. Neurology. 2014;83:e19–26.
165. Panman JL, Jiskoot LC, Bouts M, et al. Gray and white matter changes in presymptomatic genetic frontotemporal dementia: a longitudinal MRI study. Neurobiol Aging. 2019;76:115–24.
166. Rohrer JD, Nicholas JM, Cash DM, et al. Presymptomatic cognitive and neuroanatomical changes in genetic frontotemporal dementia in the genetic frontotemporal dementia initiative (GENFI) study: a cross-sectional analysis. Lancet Neurol. 2015;14:253–62.
167. Borroni B, Alberici A, Premi E, et al. Brain magnetic resonance imaging structural changes in a pedigree of asymptomatic progranulin mutation carriers. Rejuvenation Res. 2008;11:585–95.
168. Jiskoot LC, Bocchetta M, Nicholas JM, et al. Presymptomatic white matter integrity loss in familial frontotemporal dementia in the GENFI cohort: a cross-sectional diffusion tensor imaging study. Ann Clin Transl Neurol. 2018;5:1025–36.
169. Lee SE, Sias AC, Mandelli ML, et al. Network degeneration and dysfunction in presymptomatic C9ORF72 expansion carriers. Neuroimage Clin. 2017;14:286–97.

Parkinsonian Dementias

4

Contents

4.1 Parkinson's Disease and Dementia with Lewy Bodies

Parkinson's disease (PD) is a common and complex neurodegenerative disorder, mainly characterized by motor signs and symptoms, including bradykinesia, rigidity, resting tremor, and postural instability. However, the symptomatology of PD is

© Springer Nature Switzerland AG 2021
M. Filippi, F. Agosta, *Imaging Dementia*,
https://doi.org/10.1007/978-3-030-66773-3_4

now recognized as heterogeneous, with clinically significant non-motor features, involving also cognitive aspects [1]. Cognitive deficits in PD are a well-known entity, considering a clinical spectrum from subjective memory complaints to frank dementia [2, 3]. Although a condition of mild cognitive impairment (MCI) in PD could be present even at diagnosis or at early stages of disease, dementia in PD (PDD) usually occurs in advanced stages with a prevalence close to 30% [4], with an increased risk of conversion to dementia among those patients who previously had MCI [5].

Dementia with Lewy bodies (DLB) is the second most common neurodegenerative cause of dementia in older patients, after Alzheimer's disease (AD), accounting for 15–20% of cases after the age of 65 [6], and is characterized by α-synuclein aggregates as pathologic hallmarks [7]. There has been debate whether DLB and PDD are distinct disease entities or different presentations of the same underlying neurodegenerative process [8]. Although most of the DLB and PDD clinical features overlap [7], guidelines defined the 1-year rule for distinction between them according to the onset of cognitive dysfunction in relation to extrapyramidal motor symptoms (i.e., if the onset of dementia occurs within 1 year of parkinsonism, the disorder is called DLB, whereas if parkinsonism continues for more than 1 year before the onset of dementia, the disorder is called PDD) [9, 10].

4.1.1 Clinicopathological Findings

Typically, the cognitive profile observed in PDD is a dysexecutive syndrome (characterized by planning and mental flexibility deficits, and presence of apathy) with early changes including impairment of attention, visuospatial functions, slowed processing speed, and moderately impaired episodic memory [11, 12]. Significant deficits of language are not typically seen in PDD and, when present, are more likely due to the executive dysfunction-related problems rather than an intrinsic core language deficit [13]. At least one of a wide range of neuropsychiatric symptoms is reported in approximately 90% of PDD patients [14]. The most common of these symptoms are depression, hallucinations, apathy, anxiety, and insomnia, and are associated overall with excess disability, worse quality of life, poorer outcomes (in term of morbidity and mortality), and greater caregiver burden [15]. According to the current criteria, the core features of PDD are the presence of PD and a defined dementia syndrome developing within the context of established PD; the presence of specific associated cognitive and/or behavioral features allows to make a diagnosis of probable or possible PDD (Table 4.1) [16].

Similarly, DLB patients show marked deficits in executive and visuospatial/visuoperceptual functions, as well as typical cognitive fluctuations, i.e., marked variations in their level of arousal and attention during waking day. According to the current International Consensus Criteria, the core features for a diagnosis of DLB include features of parkinsonism, recurrent visual hallucinations, REM sleep behavior disorder, and cognitive fluctuations, in the context of a dementia syndrome (Table 4.2) [7]. Several additional, supportive non-motor clinical features (e.g.,

Table 4.1 Features of dementia associated with Parkinson's disease

---

I. Core features

1. Diagnosis of Parkinson's disease according to Queen Square Brain Bank criteria
2. A dementia syndrome with insidious onset and slow progression, developing within the context of established Parkinson's disease and diagnosed by history, clinical, and mental examination, defined as follows:
   - Impairment in more than one cognitive domain
   - Representing a decline from premorbid level
   - Deficits severe enough to impair daily life (social, occupational, or personal care), independent of the impairment ascribable to motor or autonomic symptoms

---

II. Associated clinical features

1. Cognitive features
   - Attention: Impaired. Impairment in spontaneous and focused attention, poor performance in attentional tasks; performance may fluctuate during the day and from day to day
   - Executive functions: Impaired. Impairment in tasks requiring initiation, planning, concept formation, rule finding, set shifting or set maintenance; impaired mental speed (bradyphrenia)
   - Visuospatial functions: Impaired. Impairment in tasks requiring visual-spatial orientation, perception, or construction
   - Memory: Impaired. Impairment in free recall of recent events or in tasks requiring learning new material, memory usually improves with cueing, recognition is usually better than free recall
   - Language: Core functions largely preserved. Word-finding difficulties and impaired comprehension of complex sentences may be present
2. Behavioral features:
   - Apathy: decreased spontaneity; loss of motivation, interest, and effortful behavior
   - Changes in personality and mood including depressive features and anxiety
   - Hallucinations: mostly visual, usually complex, formed visions of people, animals, or objects
   - Delusions: usually paranoid, such as infidelity, or phantom boarder (unwelcome guests living in the home) delusions
   - Excessive daytime sleepiness

III. Features which do not exclude PD-D, but make the diagnosis uncertain

- Coexistence of any other abnormality which may by itself cause cognitive impairment, but judged not to be the cause of dementia, e.g., presence of relevant vascular disease in imaging
- Time interval between the development of motor and cognitive symptoms not known

---

IV. Features suggesting other conditions or diseases as cause of mental impairment, which, when present make it impossible to reliably diagnose PD-D

- Cognitive and behavioral symptoms appearing solely in the context of other conditions such as the following:
  Acute confusion due to:
  a. Systemic diseases or abnormalities
  b. Drug intoxication
  Major depression according to DSM IV
- Features compatible with "probable vascular dementia" criteria according to NINDS-AIREN (dementia in the context of cerebrovascular disease as indicated by focal signs in neurological exam such as hemiparesis, sensory deficits, and evidence of relevant cerebrovascular disease by brain imaging AND a relationship between the two as indicated by the presence of one or more of the following: onset of dementia within 3 months after a recognized stroke, abrupt deterioration in cognitive functions, and fluctuating, stepwise progression of cognitive deficits).

(continued)

Table 4.1 (continued)

Criteria for the diagnosis of probable and possible PD-D

Probable PD-D

A. Core features: Both must be present

B. Associated clinical features:

- Typical profile of cognitive deficits including impairment in at least two of the four core cognitive domains (impaired attention which may fluctuate, impaired executive functions, impairment in visuospatial functions, and impaired free recall memory which usually improves with cueing)
- The presence of at least one behavioral symptom (apathy, depressed or anxious mood, hallucinations, delusions, excessive daytime sleepiness) supports the diagnosis of probable PD-D, lack of behavioral symptoms, however, does not exclude the diagnosis

C. None of the group III features present

D. None of the group IV features present

Possible PD-D

A. Core features: Both must be present

B. Associated clinical features:

- Atypical profile of cognitive impairment in one or more domains, such as prominent or receptive-type (fluent) aphasia, or pure storage-failure type amnesia (memory does not improve with cueing or in recognition tasks) with preserved attention
- Behavioral symptoms may or may not be present

OR

C. One or more of the group III features present

D. None of the group IV features present

Reproduced with permission from Emre M, Aarsland D, Brown R, et al. Clinical diagnostic criteria for dementia associated with Parkinson's disease. Movement DisordersVol. 22, No. 12, 2007, pp. 1689–1707. © 2007 Movement Disorder Society

Table 4.2 Revised criteria for the clinical diagnosis of probable and possible DLB

Essential for a diagnosis of DLB is dementia, defined as a progressive cognitive decline of sufficient magnitude to interfere with normal social or occupational functions, or with usual daily activities. Prominent or persistent memory impairment may not necessarily occur in the early stages but is usually evident with progression. Deficits on tests of attention, executive function, and visuoperceptual ability may be especially prominent and occur early.

Core clinical features (the first three typically occur early and may persist throughout the course)

Fluctuating cognition with pronounced variations in attention and alertness.

Recurrent visual hallucinations that are typically well formed and detailed.

REM sleep behavior disorder, which may precede cognitive decline.

One or more spontaneous cardinal features of parkinsonism: these are bradykinesia (defined as slowness of movement and decrement in amplitude or speed), rest tremor, or rigidity.

Supportive clinical features

Severe sensitivity to antipsychotic agents; postural instability; repeated falls; syncope or other transient episodes of unresponsiveness; severe autonomic dysfunction, e.g., constipation, orthostatic hypotension, urinary incontinence; hypersomnia; hyposmia; hallucinations in other modalities; systematized delusions; apathy, anxiety, and depression.

Indicative biomarkers

Reduced dopamine transporter uptake in basal ganglia demonstrated by SPECT or PET.

Abnormal (low uptake) [123]iodine-MIBG myocardial scintigraphy.

Polysomnographic confirmation of REM sleep without atonia.

Table 4.2   (continued)

Supportive biomarkers
Relative preservation of medial temporal lobe structures on CT/MRI scan. Generalized low uptake on SPECT/PET perfusion/metabolism scan with reduced occipital activity ± the cingulate island sign on FDG-PET imaging. Prominent posterior slow-wave activity on EEG with periodic fluctuations in the pre-alpha/theta range.
Probable DLB can be diagnosed if:
a. Two or more core clinical features of DLB are present, with or without the presence of indicative biomarkers, or b. Only one core clinical feature is present, but with one or more indicative biomarkers.
Probable DLB should not be diagnosed on the basis of biomarkers alone.
Possible DLB can be diagnosed if:
a. Only one core clinical feature of DLB is present, with no indicative biomarker evidence, or b. One or more indicative biomarkers is present, but there are no core clinical features.
DLB is less likely:
a. In the presence of any other physical illness or brain disorder including cerebrovascular disease, sufficient to account in part or in total for the clinical picture, although these do not exclude a DLB diagnosis and may serve to indicate mixed or multiple pathologies contributing to the clinical presentation, or b. If parkinsonian features are the only core clinical feature and appear for the first time at a stage of severe dementia.
DLB should be diagnosed when dementia occurs before or concurrently with parkinsonism. The term Parkinson disease dementia (PDD) should be used to describe dementia that occurs in the context of well-established Parkinson disease. In a practice setting the term that is most appropriate to the clinical situation should be used, and generic terms such as Lewy body disease are often helpful. In research studies in which distinction needs to be made between DLB and PDD, the existing 1-year rule between the onset of dementia and parkinsonism continues to be recommended.

Reproduced with permission from McKeith IG, Boeve BF, Dickson DW, et al. Diagnosis and management of dementia with Lewy bodies: Fourth consensus report of the DLB Consortium. Neurology 2017; 89:88–100. https://n.neurology.org/

autonomic dysfunction, syncope, repeated falls, delusions, depression, hypersensitivity to antipsychotic agents, etc.) are also typically reported. The presence of indicative or supportive biomarkers (some of which will be reviewed in the following paragraphs) is also important for the definition of a diagnosis of probable or possible DLB (Table 4.2) [7].

4.1.2   Neuroimaging

4.1.2.1   Structural Neuroimaging Techniques

Computed tomography (CT) and conventional magnetic resonance imaging (MRI) findings are similar in DLB and PDD, so both disorders are considered together here.

In PDD patients, CT scans can show nonspecific features, with cortical and subcortical atrophy characterized by enlarged ventricles and sulci, and abnormal caudate measures [17].

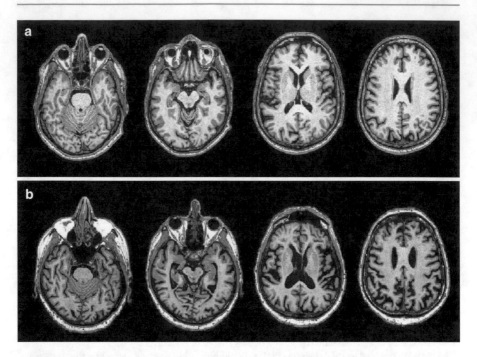

Fig. 4.1 T1-weighted MR scans of (**a**) a cognitively normal subject with Parkinson's disease (PD) and (**b**) a subject with PD associated with dementia (PDD). Global atrophy and enlarged ventricles in PDD subject are evident compared to cognitively normal patient

Conventional MRI does not reveal PD-related abnormalities in cognitively unimpaired patients, especially in the early stages, whereas with disease progression and cognitive impairment occurrence, a mild generalized atrophy with no specific topographical pattern can be observed in PDD (Fig. 4.1) and DLB patients (Fig. 4.2), together with enlargement of lateral ventricles [18]. The main clinical role of conventional MRI in these disorders is excluding other underlying pathologies such as extensive vascular disease, brain tumors, normal pressure hydrocephalus, bilateral striopallidodentate calcinosis, other potential causes of symptomatic parkinsonism (such as Wilson disease, manganese-induced parkinsonism), or different subtypes of neurodegeneration associated with brain iron accumulation, and in differentiating atypical parkinsonisms [19]. For the diagnostic workup of PDD and DLB, it is particularly important to rule out an alternative diagnosis of AD. In this view, visual inspection of T1-weighted MRI in DLB/PDD may be helpful, as it has been reported to show less atrophy in the medial temporal lobe (best assessed on coronal slices) than in AD (Fig. 4.2) (see also Chap. 1, Fig. 1.2) [20, 21]. Despite this, in both PDD and DLB, conventional structural MRI has little value for the differential diagnosis from other dementias [22].

Quantitative structural MRI studies have revealed considerable changes in gray matter in PD patients with cognitive dysfunction, showing marked atrophy in patients with dementia [23].

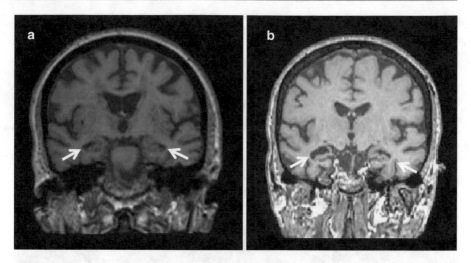

Fig. 4.2 Coronal T1-weighted images of (**a**) a patient with dementia with Lewy bodies (DLB) compared with (**b**) a patient with Alzheimer's disease (AD): the medial temporal lobes and hippocampi (arrows) appear relatively spared in DLB, supporting the differential diagnosis with AD

Whole brain atrophy in PDD has been investigated, showing a rate of atrophy of 1.12% per year in PDD patients, compared to 0.31% in non-demented PD patients and 0.34% in healthy age-matched controls [24]. On the other hand, several studies have focused on regional atrophic changes in PDD and DLB, and widespread structural changes with decreased gray matter volume have been reported, involving the frontal, temporoparietal, and occipital lobes; specifically, in PDD a major bilateral frontal atrophy has been found, whereas DLB group is characterized by a predominant parietal and occipital atrophy [25]. Interestingly, a similar involvement of subcortical regions is observed [25]. Some studies found little cortical atrophy in DLB, with only changes in the midbrain region [26], while others observed a pattern of more pronounced gray matter atrophy in the temporal, parietal, and occipital lobes in DLB compared to PDD [27], as a possible consequence of greater incidence of amyloid pathology in the former group [28].

Recent advances in structural MRI techniques, such as neuromelanin, susceptibility-weighted imaging (SWI), or iron-sensitive sequences, determine a more precise characterization of brainstem damage in PD, especially of the substantia nigra. Calbindin immunohistochemistry recognized a labeled nigral matrix and five unlabeled clusters, called nigrosomes, the largest of which (nigrosome-1) is found in the dorsal region of the substantia nigra pars compacta [29]. This structure has been observed on SWI at 3T with reduced contrast [30], and more delineated on 7T, showing a hypersignal in the axial section, in either linear or comma form and surrounded laterally and medially by a low-intensity signal, giving it a swallow tail appearance (Fig. 4.3) [31]. Recently, a meta-analysis reporting nigrosome imaging techniques showed that visual assessment of dorsolateral nigral hyperintensity provides excellent diagnostic accuracy for PD versus controls and its loss appears to be a marker of nigral pathology [32].

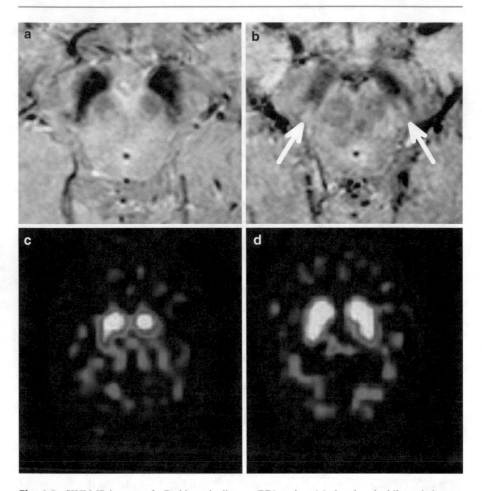

Fig. 4.3 SWI MR images of a Parkinson's disease (PD) patient (**a**) showing the bilateral absence of nigrosome-1 and a control (**b**) showing the presence of nigrosome-1 bilaterally. SPECT imaging in a PD patient shows reduction of DaT availability (**c**) compared with a healthy control (**d**). ((**a, b**) Reproduced from Schwarz ST, Afzal M, Morgan PS, et al. The 'swallow tail' appearance of the healthy nigrosome—a new accurate test of Parkinson's disease: a case-control and retrospective cross-sectional MRI study at 3T. PLoS One 2014; 9:e93814, an open-access article distributed under the terms of the Creative Commons Attribution License; (**c, d**) Reproduced from Pagano G, Niccolini F, Politis M. Imaging in Parkinson's disease. Clin Med 2016; 16:371–375)

4.1.2.2 Molecular Imaging

SPECT

PD is characterized by a progressive degeneration of the dopaminergic neurons in the substantia nigra projecting to the striatum that begins several years before clinical onset. It is estimated that the interval between onset of dopaminergic degeneration and appearance of symptoms is about 5 years, when a 40–60% neuronal loss in the substantia nigra has occurred [33]. Loss of the nigral neurons, which occurs first in the lateral layer and is then followed by the medial region, is extensive and characteristic of PD, and it leads to substantial reduction of the presynaptic dopamine transporter (DaT) [34]. Single-photon emission computed tomography (SPECT) allows objective measurement of the loss of dopaminergic function and thus is utilized in the diagnostic workup of parkinsonian syndromes (Fig. 4.3). The ^{123}I dopaminergic presynaptic ligand FP-CIT has been extensively studied in PDD/DLB and is most helpful in the differential diagnosis with AD. Abnormal FP-CIT imaging has shown good diagnostic accuracy for DLB/PDD with a specificity up to 90% for distinguishing PDD/DLB from non-DLB dementia, which is predominantly due to AD, but it is not helpful in distinguishing DLB and PDD between each other and from other parkinsonian syndromes associated with dementia (i.e., corticobasal syndrome [CBS], progressive supranuclear palsy syndrome [PSPs], and multiple system atrophy [MSA]) since nigrostriatal dopaminergic degeneration occurs in all these conditions [35]. Recently, lower ^{123}I-FP-CIT binding in the bilateral posterior putamen, but not in extrastriatal areas, in PD patients compared to DLB has been observed [36].

^{123}I-MIBG cardiac scintigraphy is widely used to assess cardiac postganglionic sympathetic degeneration, which is a common feature in neurodegenerative diseases with Lewy Bodies pathology. ^{123}I-MIBG is markedly impaired in PDD and DLB [37] and is a recommended biomarker with the ability of excluding AD and predicting conversion of possible to probable DLB with an accuracy up to 90% [38, 39].

PET

Both PDD and DLB display a widespread lateral frontal and temporoparietal hypometabolism on ^{18}F-fluorodeoxyglucose (FDG) PET, in addition to a characteristic hypometabolism of occipital cortical areas and basal ganglia, which distinguishes PDD and DLB from AD (Figs. 4.4 and 4.5) [40]. Conversely, metabolic differences between PDD and DLB appear to be subtle [40]. FDG-PET has been indicated as an important tool to identify impending PD-related cognitive decline, as patients with PDD or PD-MCI have a typical pattern of hypometabolism mainly affecting the posterior cortical areas [41]. As for DLB, the FDG-PET-based detection of the cingulate island sign, i.e., the relative preservation of mid-posterior cingulate cortex metabolism, has been included as a supportive biomarker in the diagnostic criteria for DLB (Figs. 4.4 and 4.5) [7].

Limbic and neocortical Lewy body pathology has been claimed to be the main determinant of the development of cognitive impairment in PD, whereas co-occurent cortical β-amyloid (Aβ) deposition seems to determine the rate of progression to dementia [42]. In fact, recent evidence showed that PDD patients with positive Aβ binding on ^{18}F-florbetapir PET had a faster clinical progression of dementia compared to PDD without Aβ deposits [43].

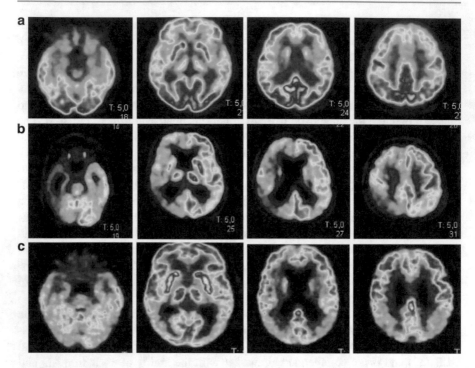

Fig. 4.4 Representative examples of FDG-PET hypometabolism pattern in patients with (**a**) progressive supranuclear palsy syndrome (PSPs), (**b**) corticobasal syndrome/corticobasal degeneration (CBS/CBD), and (**c**) Parkinson's disease associated with dementia (PDD). In PSPs, the hypometabolic pattern predominantly affects anterior cingulate, frontal-lateral cortex, striatum, the thalamus, and midbrain regions. In this case, the hypometabolism is mild and affects both hemispheres (**a**). In CBS/CBD, the most frequent FDG-PET features reported in patients with CBS is the presence of asymmetric hypometabolism in the parietal and frontal cortex, in the thalamus and ganglia of the contralateral hemispheres with respect to the most clinically affected body side. In this case, marked hypometabolism affects the right hemisphere (**b**). In patients with PDD the hypometabolic pattern includes temporoparietal and occipital cortex with spared metabolism or even relative hypermetabolism in the basal ganglia (clearly telling apart the brain metabolic profile of PDD with respect to atypical parkinsonian syndromes). As in this case (**c**), many patients with PDD are also characterized by the cingulate island sign (hypometabolism in the precuneus with relatively spared metabolism in posterior cingulate). In fact, PD, PDD, and dementia with Lewy bodies (DLB) are probably two opposite sides of the same spectrum of disease (at the moment clinically differentiated only on the basis of the timeframe of onset of cognitive and motor symptoms). (Reproduced by permission from Springer, Clinical and Translational Imaging, Role of [^{18}F]-FDG PET in patients with atypical parkinsonism associated with dementia, Raffa, S., Donegani, M.I., Borra, © 2020)

4.1.2.3 Advanced MRI Techniques

Diffusion Tensor MRI

In PDD patients, diffusion tensor (DT) MRI studies have shown lower fractional anisotropy (FA) values in the left hippocampus, bilateral anterior and posterior cingulate cortex, corpus callosum [44], as well as a more widespread global white

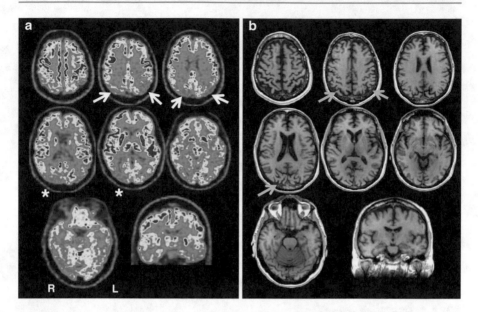

Fig. 4.5 Axial and sagittal images from (**a**) FDG-PET scan and (**b**) co-registered MRI scan of a patient with dementia with Lewy bodies, demonstrating severe hypometabolism of bilateral posterior associative cortex (white arrows), moderate hypometabolism of the right primary visual cortex (asterisks), and mild atrophy of the same regions (orange arrows). *L* left, *R* right

matter degeneration when compared to both PD and AD patients [45]. Similarly, DLB patients show extensive WM involvement, in terms of reduced FA in the corpus callosum, frontal, parietal, occipital, and temporal WM [46, 47]. Abnormalities in the occipital WM and thalamo-cortical visual pathways are characteristic findings in DLB patients [48].

Functional MRI
Functional MRI (fMRI) studies investigating brain activations in PDD have provided several data on functional connectivity abnormalities, as shown by a recent meta-analysis reporting a reduced functional brain connectivity in several brain regions involved in specific resting state networks (i.e., default mode network, auditory network, and right frontoparietal network) [49]. As for DLB, functional connectivity reductions in widespread brain regions, leading to desynchronization of cortical and subcortical areas within the attention-executive networks, have been shown to correlate with the characteristic cognitive fluctuations of this clinical presentation [50, 51]. DLB patients also display increased connectivity in the default mode network compared to AD [52], as well as reduced connectivity within motor, temporal, and frontal networks [53]. One study assessing both DLB and PDD patients reported that DLB exhibited widespread abnormalities in functional connectivity within the frontoparietal network relative to controls, while in PDD functional changes were limited to the frontal cortices and precuneus [54]. However, when comparing DLB and PDD groups there were no significant differences, suggesting only subtle functional differences between the two diseases [54].

4.2 Atypical Parkinsonisms

Atypical parkinsonisms refer to different neurodegenerative syndromes presenting with parkinsonism and clinical features that are uncommon in classical PD. The occurrence and the recognition of these signs and symptoms drive the clinician through the differential diagnosis. The main atypical parkinsonisms can be pathologically divided into tauopathies, including progressive supranuclear palsy (PSP) and corticobasal degeneration (CBD), and synucleinopathies, such as multiple system atrophy (MSA) and DLB (discussed above). An accurate differentiation between these syndromes and classical PD is important for two main reasons: first, prognosis, because life expectancy is lower in atypical parkinsonism; secondly, evaluation of treatment response, because levodopa is generally unsuccessful in atypical parkinsonism [55]. Table 4.3 shows some clinical "red flags" occurring in atypical parkinsonisms to distinguish them from PD.

4.2.1 Clinicopathological Findings

4.2.1.1 PSP Syndrome
Classically, patients with PSPs present with backward falls due to postural instability, mild symmetrical parkinsonism with predominant axial rigidity, and ocular disturbances characterized by slowed vertical saccades progressing through impaired vertical and horizontal pursuit movements to a complete ophthalmoparesis. Dementia and personality changes are common findings. Recently, new diagnostic criteria have been proposed by the Movement Disorders Society [56]: according to these, four functional domains (ocular motor dysfunction, postural instability, akinesia, and cognitive dysfunction) are identified as clinical predictors of PSP pathology. Within each domain, three clinical features representing different levels of diagnostic certainty are considered, and specific combinations of these features

Table 4.3 Red flag signs and symptoms in parkinsonism

Clinical features	Suspected diagnosis
Young onset	Juvenile PD, MSA
Axial rigidity	PSPs
Myoclonus	MSA, CBS
Vertical gaze palsy	PSPs
Early falls backward (first year)	PSPs
Asymmetric onset	PD, CBS
Alien limb/apraxia	CBS
Poor response to levodopa	PSPs, CBS, MSA
Dysautonomia	MSA
Early cognitive impairment	PSPs, CBS
Laryngeal stridor	MSA
Palilalia	PD, PSPs
Cerebellar signs	MSA
Pyramidal signs	MSA

define the diagnostic criteria, stratified by three degrees of diagnostic certainty (i.e., probable PSPs, possible PSPs, and suggestive of PSPs), and identify the clinical predominance type. Additionally, clinical clues and imaging findings were included as supportive features [56]. The cognitive profile of PSPs is characterized by prevalent attention and executive deficits, with verbal fluency severely affected (configuring, in some cases, an overlap syndrome with the nonfluent variant of primary progressive aphasia) [56], as well as deficits in both verbal and nonverbal memory with a relative preservation of recognition and with milder difficulties in construction, and naming [57]. Additionally, it has been shown that executive, language, and visuospatial abilities are generally worse than in PD and MSA, and tend to worsen over time in PSPs, but not in PD and MSA [58]; conversion to dementia was demonstrated in 16% of PSP patients after 1.5 year [58], and the only factor associated with conversion to dementia was MCI diagnosis at baseline [59].

4.2.1.2 Corticobasal Syndrome

Classical CBS is characterized by an insidious onset with progressive asymmetric levodopa-unresponsive rigidity and apraxia involving one limb. Patients with CBS show a specific neuropsychological pattern characterized by a dysexecutive syndrome, likely due to degeneration of the basal ganglia and prefrontal cortex, and asymmetric praxis disorders, which might be related to premotor and parietal lobe lesions. This neuropsychological profile may help to distinguish this condition clinically from other neurodegenerative diseases, such as PSPs or AD [60]. Other clinical phenotypes are considered on the basis of the prevalent features: frontal behavioral spatial syndrome, nonfluent/agrammatic variant of primary progressive aphasia, and PSP-CBS [61]. Indeed, CBD is a tauopathy like PSP and may have significant overlap with PSP clinical phenotypes; thus, a PSP-CBS clinical type has been identified considering the presence of ocular disturbances together with cortical and motor signs suggestive of CBD (orobuccal or limb apraxia, cortical sensory deficit, alien limb phenomena and limb rigidity, akinesia or myclonus, respectively).

4.2.1.3 Multiple System Atrophy

MSA is characterized by varying severity of parkinsonian features, cerebellar ataxia, autonomic failure, urogenital dysfunction, and corticospinal disorders. The disease frequently begins with bladder dysfunction, and, in men, erectile dysfunction. The presenting motor disorder most commonly consists of parkinsonism with bradykinesia, rigidity, and gait instability, although cerebellar ataxia is the initial motor disorder in most cases. The defining neuropathology of MSA consists of degeneration of striatonigral and olivopontocerebellar structures and the presence of cytoplasmic inclusions formed by fibrillized α-synuclein proteins. MSA can be classified into two subgroups, a cerebellar (MSA-C) and a parkinsonian (MSA-P) variant, according to the prevalent motor features [62]. Currently, cognitive dysfunction is an exclusion criterion for the diagnosis of MSA according to clinical criteria [62] and, as for PD, dementia at onset or initial stages in a patient with parkinsonism should suggest a diagnosis other than MSA, such as DLB, PSPs, or CBS. However, sparse evidence exists for some cognitive deficits in MSA. In a retrospective study on pathologically confirmed cases of 102 patients, 33 (32%) were documented to have cognitive impairment, with deficits primarily in processing speed and attention/executive functions, suggesting a frontal-subcortical pattern of dysfunction [63].

4.2.2 Neuroimaging

4.2.2.1 Structural Neuroimaging

MRI and CT scans may show generalized supratentorial atrophy in PSP, sometimes with a frontal predominance, although the most typical findings are midbrain atrophy (specifically, a thinning of the quadrigeminal plate in its superior part) and dilation of the third ventricle (Fig. 4.6) [55]. The term "hummingbird" is used to describe visual assessment of the midbrain atrophy feature on midsagittal scans, while the axial appearance has been referred to as the "Mickey Mouse" sign

Fig. 4.6 Sagittal and coronal T1-weighted MR images showing in red (1) pons and midbrain areas, as well as (2) superior cerebellar peduncle and (3) middle cerebellar peduncle widths in (**a**) a patient with progressive supranuclear palsy syndrome (PSPs) and (**b**) patient with Parkinson's disease. *PD* Parkinson's disease, *PSP-RS* PSP Richardson' syndrome. (Reproduced with permission from, Longoni G, Agosta F, Kostić VS, et al. MRI measurements of brainstem structures in patients with Richardson's syndrome, progressive supranuclear palsy-parkinsonism, and Parkinson's disease. Mov Disord 2011; 26:247–255 © 2010 Movement Disorder Society)

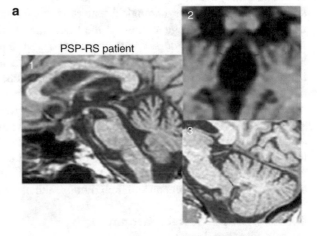

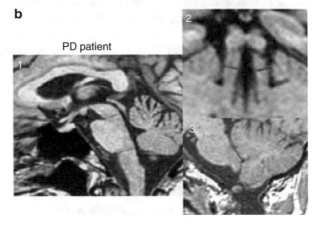

(rounded rather than rectangular midbrain peduncles) and "morning glory" sign (concavity of the lateral margin of the midbrain tegmentum) [64]. In terms of linear measurements, PSPs can be differentiated from MSA-P using a midbrain diameter <14 mm on the sagittal scan (A-P diameter) [65]. Another structure involved in PSP pathology is the superior cerebellar peduncles (SCP) due to the degeneration of dentate nucleus. Signal changes and volume reduction of SCP, with respect to middle cerebellar peduncles (MCP), could be useful in the differential diagnosis with other parkinsonian syndromes [65]. Recently, imaging biomarkers criteria for PSPs have been proposed, considering the high sensitivity and specificity for PSP diagnosis at a single-subject level of midbrain to pons ratio and magnetic resonance parkinsonism index (MRPI, i.e., [pons area/midbrain area]∗[MCP widths/SCP width]) (Fig. 4.6) [64, 66]. Other conventional imaging findings associated with PSPs are: enlargement of the third ventricle, signal increase on T2-weighted images of the midbrain and inferior olives, hypointense putamen on T2-weighted images, due to increased iron content [65].

In CBS, MRI brain findings are nonspecific but often show a characteristically asymmetric parieto-frontal cortical atrophy with "knife-like" gyri (including the pre- and post-central gyri and central sulcus) (Fig. 4.7), with less frequent involvement of the temporal lobe, and subcortical gliosis in the atrophic cortical gyri seen as high intensity on T2-weighted images. Atrophy of the corpus callosum has also been described [67]. Unfortunately, none of these MRI abnormalities is considered

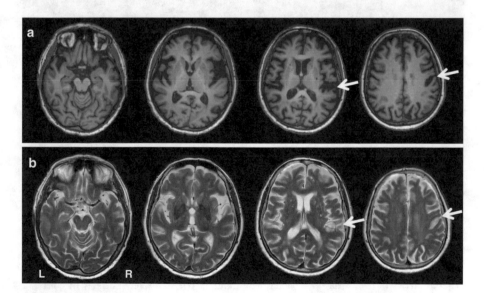

Fig. 4.7 Series of T1-weighted (**a**) and T2-weighted (**b**) MR images of a patient diagnosed with corticobasal syndrome, showing atrophy of the posterior frontal and parietal lobes with a right-sided predominance (arrows). *L* left, *R* right

to be of clearly diagnostic or even pathognomonic relevance for CBS, mainly due to the pathological heterogeneity of this syndrome [68].

A number of conventional MRI findings have been described as suggestive of MSA. These include: postero-lateral putaminal decreased signal intensity on T2-weighted images, covered by a rim of increased signal, mainly due to iron deposition and gliosis, respectively; a cruciform linear area of high signal on T2-weighted images in the pons, also known as "hot-cross bun" sign, which is typically associated with MSA-C and is produced by the selective loss of myelinated transverse pontocerebellar fibers and neurons in the pontine raphe, with relative preservation of the pontine tegmentum and corticospinal tracts (Fig. 4.8); cerebellar and pontine atrophy with hyperintensity and atrophy of the MCP [69]. A summary of MRI features in atypical parkinsonisms is provided in Table 4.4.

Quantitative structural MRI studies have shown gray matter loss in midbrain, frontal lobes, supplemental motor area, caudate nucleus, thalamus, cerebellar lobes, and dentate nuclei in PSPs patients compared to healthy controls and other

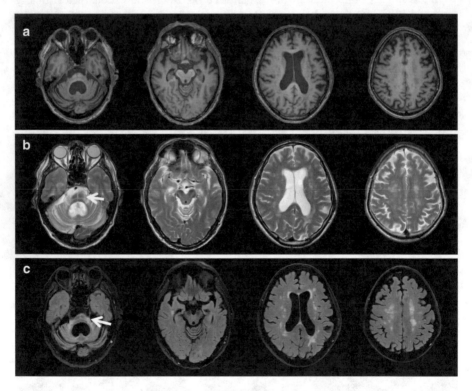

Fig. 4.8 Series of MRI scans of a patient with multiple system atrophy. Atrophy of pons and middle cerebellar peduncles is one of the main finding on T1-weighted images (**a**). A widespread atrophy is also visible. Typical cruciform linear hyperintensity (hot-cross bun sign) is seen in the pons, especially on T2-weighted (**b**) and FLAIR (**c**) axial MR images (arrows)

Table 4.4 MRI features in atypical parkinsonian syndromes [107]

	MRI sequence	Imaging features	Discriminates
Progressive supranuclear palsy syndrome (PSPs)	T1 sagittal	Midbrain atrophy (AP diameter <14 mm)	PSP from MSA
	T1 sagittal	Concave upper midbrain border	PSP from PD
	T1 coronal	SCP atrophy	PSP from MSA, PD
	T1 sagittal	Ratio of midbrain/pons—"hummingbird"	PSP from MSA
Multiple system atrophy (MSA)	T2 axial	"Hot cross bun"	MSAc from PSP, PD
	T2 axial	Putamen hypointensity	MSA from PD
	T2 axial	Putamen slit sign	MSAp from PSP, PD
Corticobasal degeneration syndrome (CBS)	T1	Global atrophy	Seen in advanced PSP
	T1	Asymmetric cortical atrophy	Suggestive of CBD

Reproduced with permission from Barkhof F, Fox NC, Bastos-Leite AJ, Scheltens P. Neuroimaging in Dementia. Springer-Verlag Berlin Heidelberg, 2011

parkinsonian syndromes [70–72], suggesting that not only visual inspection of conventional MRI but also advanced techniques, including VBM analysis, can provide clues to evaluate these diverse atrophic changes [73]. A meta-analysis study showed that PSPs exhibits significant convergence for gray matter reduction in the medial thalamus, which was described in 58% of studies. This was the largest cluster, with extension to the midbrain. The bilateral insula, left caudate, and medial frontal gyrus were also involved [74].

In CBS, VBM studies showed a more prominent asymmetric atrophy in the frontoparietal cortex and in the basal ganglia, with focal atrophy of premotor and supplemental motor areas [74, 75]; additionally, reduced cortical thickness in the frontoparietal regions contralateral to the clinically more affected side has been shown to be a more sensitive measure than volumetric changes [76]. In the comparison with PSPs patients, CBS showed a pattern of cortical atrophy involving dorsal frontal and parietal cortices, while midbrain structures were more atrophic in PSPs [77].

In MSA-P patients compared to controls, selective cortical atrophy involving the primary motor areas, prefrontal cortex, and insula was identified by means of VBM techniques [78], and a different pattern and localization of gray matter reduction involving putamen and claustrum was identified in the MSA-P in comparison with PD [79]. Very recently, it has been demonstrated that MSA-p patients, showing multidomain cognitive impairment, exhibit significant cortical thinning of frontotemporal–parietal regions and atrophy of periaqueductal gray matter, left cerebellar hemisphere, left pallidum and bilateral putamen, compared to controls [80]. Moreover, cortical thinning in temporal regions correlated with global cognitive status and memory impairment [80].

4.2.2.2 Molecular Imaging

SPECT and PET tracers investigating presynaptic dopaminergic function cannot differentiate PD from atypical parkinsonisms, due to a similar nigrostriatal involvement in these conditions, although asymmetry of binding loss tends to be more pronounced in PD. Evaluation of presynaptic dopaminergic function in PSPs patients with PET with F-DOPA revealed severe bilateral reductions of uptake in the caudate and the anterior and posterior putamen, compared with PD [81]. Considering neuronal cell metabolism, FDG-PET can discriminate PSPs from PD, showing hypometabolism in the frontal lobes, anterior cingulate cortex, and also in the midbrain, and may be useful in early stages of the disease, when the clinical diagnosis is less certain (Fig. 4.4) [82]. As for CBS, the pattern of metabolic abnormalities consists of a decreased FDG uptake, which is mainly contralateral to the side of prominent symptoms with a predominance in the parietotemporal, prefrontal, cingular, and motor cortices, and balanced involvement of caudate and putamen (Figs. 4.4 and 4.9). The occipital cortex and cerebellum are usually spared. Differential diagnosis between CBS and other atypical parkinsonisms using FDG-PET show a good sensitivity (81–91%) and specificity (91–100%) [83]. A very recent study investigating different patterns of metabolism considering post-mortem neuropathological diagnosis of patients suggested that FDG-PET could be useful in the differential diagnosis of CBS spectrum [41]. They found in the whole CBS group, compared to healthy controls, a significant hypometabolism in frontoparietal regions, including the perirolandic area, basal ganglia, and thalamus of the clinically more affected hemisphere. Patients with CBS-CBD showed a similar pattern with a more prominent, bilateral involvement of the basal ganglia. Patients with CBS-AD presented with posterior, asymmetric hypometabolism, including the lateral parietal and temporal lobes and the posterior cingulate. Finally, CBS-PSP patients exhibited a more anterior hypometabolic pattern, including the medial frontal regions and the anterior cingulate [41].

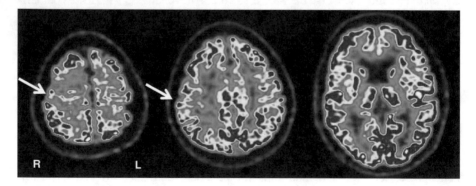

Fig. 4.9 Axial images from the FDG-PET scan of a patient with corticobasal syndrome, demonstrating mild hypometabolism of posterior frontal regions in the right hemisphere (arrows). *L* left, *R* right

Regarding MSA, PET with F-DOPA cannot be used in the clinical setting to differentiate MSA from PD due to the overlap of binding pattern, even if it could show a more prominent bilateral binding reduction [81]. On the other hand, FP-CIT uptake was found to be more reduced in the ventral putamen earlier than PD patients [84], and differences in FP-CIT uptake seemed to be related to different subtypes of MSA showing that MSA-P or mixed features exhibited more severe DaT loss in the striatum compared to MSA-C [84]. FDG-PET shows bilateral hypometabolism of the putamen, brainstem, and cerebellum in MSA, and this pattern, highly reproducible across studies, has been included as supportive criteria for MSA diagnosis [62].

As mentioned in the "Parkinson's disease and dementia with Lewy body" section, ^{123}I-MIBG uptake is markedly reduced in DLB and PDD patients, and could be a useful tool for differentiating DLB from other parkinsonian syndromes with dementia, such as PSPs and CBS. As for MSA, the main responsible lesions for cardiovascular autonomic dysfunction are the brainstem and preganglionic sympathetic nerves, preserving postganglionic terminals and leading to a normal MIBG uptake [85].

4.2.2.3 Advanced MRI Techniques

Diffusion Tensor MRI

Diffusion tensor (DT) MRI analysis in PSPs patients compared to healthy controls showed significantly reduced FA in SCP, body of the corpus callosum, regions of the superior longitudinal fasciculus in the posterior frontal lobes, inferior longitudinal fasciculus, thalamus, cingulum, and fornix [71, 86, 87]. Moreover, white matter measures were found to be highly associated with cognitive deficits in PSPs [87]. The comparison between PSPs and CBS showed overlapping regions of reduced FA and increased MD in the body of the corpus callosum, middle cingulum bundle, and premotor and prefrontal white matter, with reduced FA also observed in the SCP in both syndromes. On the other hand, CBS patients showed a supratentorial and asymmetric posterior pattern of degeneration with greater involvement of the splenium of the corpus callosum, premotor, motor, and parietal lobes. Conversely, PSPs showed a more symmetric and infratentorial pattern of degeneration, with greater involvement of the SCP and midbrain, suggesting the involvement of a common structural network with subtle differences that could be used as biomarkers for differentiating these two syndromes [88]. Discrimination between CBS, PSPs, and PD patients was assessed using a hemispheric symmetry ratio obtained by apparent diffusion coefficient (ADC) maps [89]. The hemispheric symmetry ratio differentiated CBS patients from PSPa and PD with a sensitivity and specificity of 100% [89].

As for MSA, diffusivity measures of the MCP discriminated MSA-P from PD with a sensitivity and specificity of 100% [90]. A recent meta-analysis on DWI in MSA showed an overall sensitivity of 90% and an overall specificity of 93% to distinguish MSA-P from PD based on putaminal diffusivity [91]. Furthermore, putaminal diffusivity measures were more accurate in discriminating MSA-P from PD as compared with SPECT with IBZM (another DaT-binding tracer) [92], cardiac

MIBG [93], and FDG-PET imaging [94]. A DT MRI study examined patients with movement disorders with a multitarget imaging approach focused on the basal ganglia and cerebellum and accurately classified PD patients versus MSA (94% sensitivity, 100% specificity), and MSA versus PSP (90% sensitivity, 100% specificity) [95].

Functional MRI

Resting-state fMRI has been applied to patients with PSPs, who showed resting state functional connectivity disruptions within a cortico-subcortical and cortico-brainstem network, involved in motor, oculomotor, and cognitive functions [96–99]. A significant inverse correlation between midbrain-associated network connectivity activation and disease stage was found [99], and reduced functional connectivity between thalamic, basal ganglia, and cortical structures correlated with measures of cognitive dysfunction [71, 96]. Decreased functional connectivity within the default mode network, involving prefrontal cortex, has also been correlated with worse cognitive performance [98]. A longitudinal assessment of PSPs patients showed that patients with more severe baseline impairment had greater subsequent prefrontal-parietal cortical functional connectivity decline, while patients with more rapid longitudinal clinical decline showed decreased functional connectivity in the prefrontal-paralimbic system [97].

Patients with CBS have shown increased within-network connectivity, compared with healthy controls, highlighting a global hyperconnectivity in brain regions related to motor and cognitive/affective functions, as a possible compensation mechanism due to a plasticity-related shift in neuronal activity from atrophic to intact brain structures or as a direct consequence of disrupted neuronal activity caused by neurodegeneration [100]. A recent study found an increased functional connectivity between the dentate nucleus and the sensorimotor cortex, contralateral to the most clinically affected side, suggesting an unbalanced reorganization of cerebellum connections secondary to asymmetric motor and higher cortical symptoms [101].

During resting state fMRI, compared to healthy controls, MSA patients showed decreased default mode network connectivity [102], as well as decreased connectivity in several cerebellar, pontine, and temporoparietal cortical regions, with strong correlation between functional connectivity and clinical performance [103]. In addition, the degrees of connectivity from the right dentate nucleus to the right cerebellum negatively correlated with Unified Parkinson's Disease Rating Scale-III scores in patients with MSA, while showing a positive association with Montreal Cognitive Assessment scores; these findings suggest different mechanisms of cerebellar functional activity responsible for motor and cognitive impairment in this condition [104]. Cognitive deficits in MSA were also suggested to be driven by decreased cerebello-prefrontal and cerebello-amygdaloid functional connections [105].

4.3   Clinical Case #1

A 78-year-old male patient presents with a 4-year history of cognitive and neuropsychiatric complaints, characterized by progressive decline in attention and memory, severe mood depression, and anxiety. As reported by his caregivers, despite a general worsening of these symptoms over time, there are still some days or hours of the day (particularly, morning hours) when the patient seems "unexpectedly normal" from a cognitive point of view. In the last 2 years, the patient also presented evidence of flexed posture and bradykinesia in his gait, together with alterations of his handwriting, which became micrographic. During the last few months, frequent awakenings and episodes of confusion have occurred during the night. For this reason, an antipsychotic treatment with promazine was initiated, and then soon discontinued due to the occurrence of visual hallucinations. He underwent brain MRI, which showed diffuse brain atrophy, with a more salient widening of parietal sulci and relative sparing of the medial temporal lobe structures (Fig. 4.10), in the absence of significant vascular pathology. FP-CIT SPECT showed severe depletion of dopaminergic synaptic terminals in the putamina, bilaterally. A diagnosis of probable DLB, based on clinical criteria and the presence of two supportive biomarkers, was made.

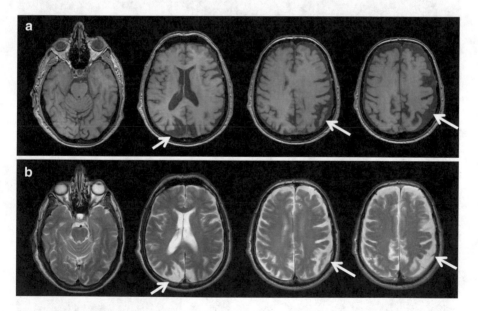

Fig. 4.10 Series of T1-weighted (**a**) and T2-weighted (**b**) MR images of a patient diagnosed with probable dementia with Lewy bodies (clinical case #1). Scans show diffuse brain atrophy, with a more salient widening of occipital and parietal sulci (arrows) and relative sparing of the medial temporal lobe structures, in the absence of significant vascular pathology. The atrophy is better appreciated on T1-weighted scans (**a**)

4.4   Clinical Case #2

A 55-year-old right-handed lady presented to medical attention complaining a 2-year history of speech output difficulties, particularly when articulating complex words or syllables. During the last months, she also noticed some clumsiness when using the left hand for manipulating objects. Neurological examination showed a left-sided mild extrapyramidal bradykinetic-rigid syndrome, as well as orobuccal and right limb apraxia. Language assessment demonstrated the presence of prominent speech output impairment and mild agrammatism. Analyses of FDG PET and structural MRI (Fig. 4.11) showed right greater than left frontal hypometabolism and atrophy, including the Broca's area. A functional MRI scan performed during a naming task demonstrated bilateral language activations in the patient's brain, despite her right-handedness. DaT-scan showed a reduced uptake in the right striatum. Based on current criteria [61], the patient was diagnosed with probable CBS with a co-occurrent presentation of "crossed" nonfluent/agrammatic variant of primary progressive aphasia (nfvPPA). See Ref. [106] for further details regarding this case.

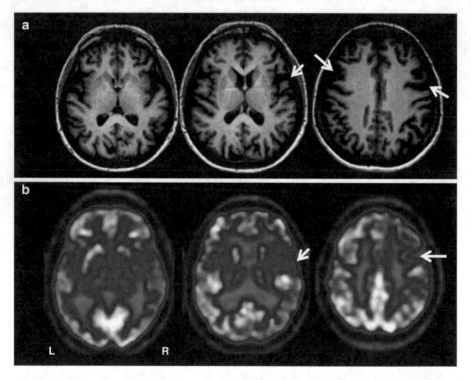

Fig. 4.11 T1-weighted MR scan (**a**) and FDG-PET scan (**b**) of patient with probable CBS with a co-occurrent presentation of nonfluent/agrammatic variant of primary progressive aphasia (crossed variant, clinical case #2). Scans show right greater than left frontal hypometabolism and damage (arrows), including the Broca's area. (Reproduced by permission from Springer, Journal of Neurology, A multimodal neuroimaging study of a case of crossed nonfluent/agrammatic primary progressive aphasia, Spinelli EG, Caso F, Agosta F, et al. © 2015)

References

1. Kalia LV, Lang AE. Parkinson's disease. Lancet. 2015;386:896–912.
2. Monastero R, Cicero CE, Baschi R, et al. Mild cognitive impairment in Parkinson's disease: the Parkinson's disease cognitive study (PACOS). J Neurol. 2018;265:1050–8.
3. Baschi R, Nicoletti A, Restivo V, et al. Frequency and correlates of subjective memory complaints in Parkinson's disease with and without mild cognitive impairment: data from the Parkinson's disease cognitive impairment study. J Alzheimers Dis. 2018;63:1015–24.
4. Aarsland D, Creese B, Politis M, et al. Cognitive decline in Parkinson disease. Nat Rev Neurol. 2017;13:217–31.
5. Nicoletti A, Luca A, Baschi R, et al. Incidence of mild cognitive impairment and dementia in Parkinson's disease: the Parkinson's disease cognitive impairment study. Front Aging Neurosci. 2019;11:21.
6. Taylor JP, O'Brien J. Neuroimaging of dementia with Lewy bodies. Neuroimaging Clin N Am. 2012;22:67–81, viii.
7. McKeith IG, Boeve BF, Dickson DW, et al. Diagnosis and management of dementia with Lewy bodies: fourth consensus report of the DLB consortium. Neurology. 2017;89:88–100.
8. Aarsland D, Ballard CG, Halliday G. Are Parkinson's disease with dementia and dementia with Lewy bodies the same entity? J Geriatr Psychiatry Neurol. 2004;17:137–45.
9. Lippa CF, Duda JE, Grossman M, et al. DLB and PDD boundary issues: diagnosis, treatment, molecular pathology, and biomarkers. Neurology. 2007;68:812–9.
10. Klein JC, Eggers C, Kalbe E, et al. Neurotransmitter changes in dementia with Lewy bodies and Parkinson disease dementia in vivo. Neurology. 2010;74:885–92.
11. Fields JA. Cognitive and neuropsychiatric features in Parkinson's and Lewy body dementias. Arch Clin Neuropsychol. 2017;32:786–801.
12. Hanagasi HA, Tufekcioglu Z, Emre M. Dementia in Parkinson's disease. J Neurol Sci. 2017;374:26–31.
13. Grossman M, Gross RG, Moore P, et al. Difficulty processing temporary syntactic ambiguities in Lewy body spectrum disorder. Brain Lang. 2012;120:52–60.
14. Aarsland D, Bronnick K, Ehrt U, et al. Neuropsychiatric symptoms in patients with Parkinson's disease and dementia: frequency, profile and associated care giver stress. J Neurol Neurosurg Psychiatry. 2007;78:36–42.
15. Weintraub D, Mamikonyan E. The neuropsychiatry of Parkinson disease: a perfect storm. Am J Geriatr Psychiatry. 2019;27:998–1018.
16. Emre M, Aarsland D, Brown R, et al. Clinical diagnostic criteria for dementia associated with Parkinson's disease. Mov Disord. 2007;22:1689–707; quiz 1837.
17. Inzelberg R, Treves T, Reider I, Gerlenter I, Korczyn AD. Computed tomography brain changes in parkinsonian dementia. Neuroradiology. 1987;29:535–9.
18. Camicioli R, Sabino J, Gee M, et al. Ventricular dilatation and brain atrophy in patients with Parkinson's disease with incipient dementia. Mov Disord. 2011;26:1443–50.
19. Seppi K, Poewe W. Brain magnetic resonance imaging techniques in the diagnosis of parkinsonian syndromes. Neuroimaging Clin N Am. 2010;20:29–55.
20. Nedelska Z, Ferman TJ, Boeve BF, et al. Pattern of brain atrophy rates in autopsy-confirmed dementia with Lewy bodies. Neurobiol Aging. 2015;36:452–61.
21. Silbert LC, Kaye J. Neuroimaging and cognition in Parkinson's disease dementia. Brain Pathol. 2010;20:646–53.
22. Walker Z, Possin KL, Boeve BF, Aarsland D. Lewy body dementias. Lancet. 2015;386:1683–97.
23. Hall JM, Lewis SJG. Neural correlates of cognitive impairment in Parkinson's disease: a review of structural MRI findings. Int Rev Neurobiol. 2019;144:1–28.
24. Burton EJ, McKeith IG, Burn DJ, Williams ED, O'Brien JT. Cerebral atrophy in Parkinson's disease with and without dementia: a comparison with Alzheimer's disease, dementia with Lewy bodies and controls. Brain. 2004;127:791–800.

25. Borroni B, Premi E, Formenti A, et al. Structural and functional imaging study in dementia with Lewy bodies and Parkinson's disease dementia. Parkinsonism Relat Disord. 2015;21:1049–55.
26. Watson R, Blamire AM, O'Brien JT. Magnetic resonance imaging in lewy body dementias. Dement Geriatr Cogn Disord. 2009;28:493–506.
27. Beyer MK, Larsen JP, Aarsland D. Gray matter atrophy in Parkinson disease with dementia and dementia with Lewy bodies. Neurology. 2007;69:747–54.
28. Mak E, Su L, Williams GB, O'Brien JT. Neuroimaging characteristics of dementia with Lewy bodies. Alzheimers Res Ther. 2014;6:18.
29. Arribarat G, De Barros A, Peran P. Modern brainstem MRI techniques for the diagnosis of Parkinson's disease and Parkinsonisms. Front Neurol. 2020;11:791.
30. Gao P, Zhou PY, Li G, et al. Visualization of nigrosomes-1 in 3T MR susceptibility weighted imaging and its absence in diagnosing Parkinson's disease. Eur Rev Med Pharmacol Sci. 2015;19:4603–9.
31. Cosottini M, Frosini D, Pesaresi I, et al. MR imaging of the substantia nigra at 7 T enables diagnosis of Parkinson disease. Radiology. 2014;271:831–8.
32. Mahlknecht P, Krismer F, Poewe W, Seppi K. Meta-analysis of dorsolateral nigral hyperintensity on magnetic resonance imaging as a marker for Parkinson's disease. Mov Disord. 2017;32:619–23.
33. Cummings JL, Henchcliffe C, Schaier S, et al. The role of dopaminergic imaging in patients with symptoms of dopaminergic system neurodegeneration. Brain. 2011;134:3146–66.
34. Palermo G, Ceravolo R. Molecular imaging of the dopamine transporter. Cells. 2019;8:872.
35. McKeith I, O'Brien J, Walker Z, et al. Sensitivity and specificity of dopamine transporter imaging with 123I-FP-CIT SPECT in dementia with Lewy bodies: a phase III, multicentre study. Lancet Neurol. 2007;6:305–13.
36. Joling M, Vriend C, van der Zande JJ, et al. Lower (123)I-FP-CIT binding to the striatal dopamine transporter, but not to the extrastriatal serotonin transporter, in Parkinson's disease compared with dementia with Lewy bodies. Neuroimage Clin. 2018;19:130–6.
37. Oka H, Yoshioka M, Morita M, et al. Reduced cardiac 123I-MIBG uptake reflects cardiac sympathetic dysfunction in Lewy body disease. Neurology. 2007;69:1460–5.
38. Oda H, Ishii K, Terashima A, et al. Myocardial scintigraphy may predict the conversion to probable dementia with Lewy bodies. Neurology. 2013;81:1741–5.
39. Chételat G, Arbizu J, Barthel H, et al. Amyloid-PET and ^{18}F-FDG-PET in the diagnostic investigation of Alzheimer's disease and other dementias. Lancet Neurol. 2020;19:951.
40. Meyer PT, Frings L, Rucker G, Hellwig S. (18)F-FDG PET in parkinsonism: differential diagnosis and evaluation of cognitive impairment. J Nucl Med. 2017;58:1888–98.
41. Pardini M, Huey ED, Spina S, et al. FDG-PET patterns associated with underlying pathology in corticobasal syndrome. Neurology. 2019;92:e1121–35.
42. Compta Y, Parkkinen L, O'Sullivan SS, et al. Lewy- and Alzheimer-type pathologies in Parkinson's disease dementia: which is more important? Brain. 2011;134:1493–505.
43. Palermo G, Tommasini L, Aghakhanyan G, et al. Clinical correlates of cerebral amyloid deposition in Parkinson's disease dementia: evidence from a PET study. J Alzheimers Dis. 2019;70:597–609.
44. Bledsoe IO, Stebbins GT, Merkitch D, Goldman JG. White matter abnormalities in the corpus callosum with cognitive impairment in Parkinson disease. Neurology. 2018;91:e2244–55.
45. Perea RD, Rada RC, Wilson J, et al. A comparative white matter study with Parkinson's disease, Parkinson's disease with dementia and Alzheimer's disease. J Alzheimers Dis Parkinsonism. 2013;3:123.
46. Nedelska Z, Schwarz CG, Boeve BF, et al. White matter integrity in dementia with Lewy bodies: a voxel-based analysis of diffusion tensor imaging. Neurobiol Aging. 2015;36:2010–7.
47. Lee JE, Park HJ, Park B, et al. A comparative analysis of cognitive profiles and white-matter alterations using voxel-based diffusion tensor imaging between patients with Parkinson's disease dementia and dementia with Lewy bodies. J Neurol Neurosurg Psychiatry. 2010;81:320–6.

48. Delli Pizzi S, Maruotti V, Taylor JP, et al. Relevance of subcortical visual pathways disruption to visual symptoms in dementia with Lewy bodies. Cortex. 2014;59:12–21.
49. Wolters AF, van de Weijer SCF, Leentjens AFG, et al. Resting-state fMRI in Parkinson's disease patients with cognitive impairment: a meta-analysis. Parkinsonism Relat Disord. 2019;62:16–27.
50. Lowther ER, O'Brien JT, Firbank MJ, Blamire AM. Lewy body compared with Alzheimer dementia is associated with decreased functional connectivity in resting state networks. Psychiatry Res. 2014;223:192–201.
51. Peraza LR, Kaiser M, Firbank M, et al. fMRI resting state networks and their association with cognitive fluctuations in dementia with Lewy bodies. Neuroimage Clin. 2014;4:558–65.
52. Franciotti R, Falasca NW, Bonanni L, et al. Default network is not hypoactive in dementia with fluctuating cognition: an Alzheimer disease/dementia with Lewy bodies comparison. Neurobiol Aging. 2013;34:1148–58.
53. Schumacher J, Peraza LR, Firbank M, et al. Functional connectivity in dementia with Lewy bodies: a within- and between-network analysis. Hum Brain Mapp. 2018;39:1118–29.
54. Peraza LR, Colloby SJ, Firbank MJ, et al. Resting state in Parkinson's disease dementia and dementia with Lewy bodies: commonalities and differences. Int J Geriatr Psychiatry. 2015;30:1135–46.
55. Wenning GK, Litvan I, Tolosa E. Milestones in atypical and secondary Parkinsonisms. Mov Disord. 2011;26:1083–95.
56. Hoglinger GU, Respondek G, Stamelou M, et al. Clinical diagnosis of progressive supranuclear palsy: the movement disorder society criteria. Mov Disord. 2017;32:853–64.
57. Gerstenecker A, Mast B, Duff K, et al. Executive dysfunction is the primary cognitive impairment in progressive supranuclear palsy. Arch Clin Neuropsychol. 2013;28:104–13.
58. Fiorenzato E, Antonini A, Camparini V, et al. Characteristics and progression of cognitive deficits in progressive supranuclear palsy vs. multiple system atrophy and Parkinson's disease. J Neural Transm (Vienna). 2019;126:1437–45.
59. Pilotto A, Gazzina S, Benussi A, et al. Mild cognitive impairment and progression to dementia in progressive supranuclear palsy. Neurodegener Dis. 2017;17:286–91.
60. Pillon B, Blin J, Vidailhet M, et al. The neuropsychological pattern of corticobasal degeneration: comparison with progressive supranuclear palsy and Alzheimer's disease. Neurology. 1995;45:1477–83.
61. Armstrong MJ, Litvan I, Lang AE, et al. Criteria for the diagnosis of corticobasal degeneration. Neurology. 2013;80:496–503.
62. Gilman S, Wenning GK, Low PA, et al. Second consensus statement on the diagnosis of multiple system atrophy. Neurology. 2008;71:670–6.
63. Koga S, Parks A, Uitti RJ, et al. Profile of cognitive impairment and underlying pathology in multiple system atrophy. Mov Disord. 2017;32:405–13.
64. Whitwell JL, Hoglinger GU, Antonini A, et al. Radiological biomarkers for diagnosis in PSP: where are we and where do we need to be? Mov Disord. 2017;32:955–71.
65. Schrag A, Good CD, Miszkiel K, et al. Differentiation of atypical parkinsonian syndromes with routine MRI. Neurology. 2000;54:697–702.
66. Quattrone A, Nicoletti G, Messina D, et al. MR imaging index for differentiation of progressive supranuclear palsy from Parkinson disease and the Parkinson variant of multiple system atrophy. Radiology. 2008;246:214–21.
67. Savoiardo M. Differential diagnosis of Parkinson's disease and atypical parkinsonian disorders by magnetic resonance imaging. Neurol Sci. 2003;24(Suppl 1):S35–7.
68. Heim B, Krismer F, Seppi K. Structural imaging in atypical parkinsonism. Int Rev Neurobiol. 2018;142:67–148.
69. Krismer F, Seppi K, Wenning GK, et al. Abnormalities on structural MRI associate with faster disease progression in multiple system atrophy. Parkinsonism Relat Disord. 2019;58:23–7.
70. Shi HC, Zhong JG, Pan PL, et al. Gray matter atrophy in progressive supranuclear palsy: meta-analysis of voxel-based morphometry studies. Neurol Sci. 2013;34:1049–55.

71. Whitwell JL, Avula R, Master A, et al. Disrupted thalamocortical connectivity in PSP: a resting-state fMRI, DTI, and VBM study. Parkinsonism Relat Disord. 2011;17:599–605.
72. Agosta F, Kostic VS, Galantucci S, et al. The in vivo distribution of brain tissue loss in Richardson's syndrome and PSP-parkinsonism: a VBM-DARTEL study. Eur J Neurosci. 2010;32:640–7.
73. Sakurai K, Tokumaru AM, Shimoji K, et al. Beyond the midbrain atrophy: wide spectrum of structural MRI finding in cases of pathologically proven progressive supranuclear palsy. Neuroradiology. 2017;59:431–43.
74. Yu F, Barron DS, Tantiwongkosi B, Fox P. Patterns of gray matter atrophy in atypical parkinsonism syndromes: a VBM meta-analysis. Brain Behav. 2015;5:e00329.
75. Whitwell JL, Jack CR Jr, Boeve BF, et al. Imaging correlates of pathology in corticobasal syndrome. Neurology. 2010;75:1879–87.
76. Upadhyay N, Suppa A, Piattella MC, et al. Gray and white matter structural changes in corticobasal syndrome. Neurobiol Aging. 2016;37:82–90.
77. Boxer AL, Geschwind MD, Belfor N, et al. Patterns of brain atrophy that differentiate corticobasal degeneration syndrome from progressive supranuclear palsy. Arch Neurol. 2006;63:81–6.
78. Brenneis C, Seppi K, Schocke MF, et al. Voxel-based morphometry detects cortical atrophy in the Parkinson variant of multiple system atrophy. Mov Disord. 2003;18:1132–8.
79. Shao N, Yang J, Shang H. Voxelwise meta-analysis of gray matter anomalies in Parkinson variant of multiple system atrophy and Parkinson's disease using anatomic likelihood estimation. Neurosci Lett. 2015;587:79–86.
80. Caso F, Canu E, Lukic MJ, et al. Cognitive impairment and structural brain damage in multiple system atrophy-parkinsonian variant. J Neurol. 2020;267:87–94.
81. Brooks DJ, Ibanez V, Sawle GV, et al. Differing patterns of striatal 18F-dopa uptake in Parkinson's disease, multiple system atrophy, and progressive supranuclear palsy. Ann Neurol. 1990;28:547–55.
82. Xu Z, Arbizu J, Pavese N. PET molecular imaging in atypical parkinsonism. Int Rev Neurobiol. 2018;142:3–36.
83. Walker Z, Gandolfo F, Orini S, et al. Clinical utility of FDG PET in Parkinson's disease and atypical parkinsonism associated with dementia. Eur J Nucl Med Mol Imaging. 2018;45:1534–45.
84. Oh M, Kim JS, Kim JY, et al. Subregional patterns of preferential striatal dopamine transporter loss differ in Parkinson disease, progressive supranuclear palsy, and multiple-system atrophy. J Nucl Med. 2012;53:399–406.
85. Orimo S, Yogo M, Nakamura T, Suzuki M, Watanabe H. (123)I-meta-iodobenzylguanidine (MIBG) cardiac scintigraphy in alpha-synucleinopathies. Ageing Res Rev. 2016;30:122–33.
86. Canu E, Agosta F, Baglio F, et al. Diffusion tensor magnetic resonance imaging tractography in progressive supranuclear palsy. Mov Disord. 2011;26:1752–5.
87. Caso F, Agosta F, Volonte MA, et al. Cognitive impairment in progressive supranuclear palsy-Richardson's syndrome is related to white matter damage. Parkinsonism Relat Disord. 2016;31:65–71.
88. Whitwell JL, Schwarz CG, Reid RI, et al. Diffusion tensor imaging comparison of progressive supranuclear palsy and corticobasal syndromes. Parkinsonism Relat Disord. 2014;20:493–8.
89. Rizzo G, Martinelli P, Manners D, et al. Diffusion-weighted brain imaging study of patients with clinical diagnosis of corticobasal degeneration, progressive supranuclear palsy and Parkinson's disease. Brain. 2008;131:2690–700.
90. Nicoletti G, Lodi R, Condino F, et al. Apparent diffusion coefficient measurements of the middle cerebellar peduncle differentiate the Parkinson variant of MSA from Parkinson's disease and progressive supranuclear palsy. Brain. 2006;129:2679–87.
91. Bajaj S, Krismer F, Palma JA, et al. Diffusion-weighted MRI distinguishes Parkinson disease from the parkinsonian variant of multiple system atrophy: a systematic review and meta-analysis. PLoS One. 2017;12:e0189897.

92. Seppi K, Schocke MF, Donnemiller E, et al. Comparison of diffusion-weighted imaging and [123I]IBZM-SPECT for the differentiation of patients with the Parkinson variant of multiple system atrophy from those with Parkinson's disease. Mov Disord. 2004;19:1438–45.

93. Kollensperger M, Seppi K, Liener C, et al. Diffusion weighted imaging best discriminates PD from MSA-P: a comparison with tilt table testing and heart MIBG scintigraphy. Mov Disord. 2007;22:1771–6.

94. Baudrexel S, Seifried C, Penndorf B, et al. The value of putaminal diffusion imaging versus 18-fluorodeoxyglucose positron emission tomography for the differential diagnosis of the Parkinson variant of multiple system atrophy. Mov Disord. 2014;29:380–7.

95. Prodoehl J, Li H, Planetta PJ, et al. Diffusion tensor imaging of Parkinson's disease, atypical parkinsonism, and essential tremor. Mov Disord. 2013;28:1816–22.

96. Piattella MC, Tona F, Bologna M, et al. Disrupted resting-state functional connectivity in progressive supranuclear palsy. AJNR Am J Neuroradiol. 2015;36:915–21.

97. Brown JA, Hua AY, Trujllo A, et al. Advancing functional dysconnectivity and atrophy in progressive supranuclear palsy. Neuroimage Clin. 2017;16:564–74.

98. Rosskopf J, Gorges M, Muller HP, et al. Intrinsic functional connectivity alterations in progressive supranuclear palsy: differential effects in frontal cortex, motor, and midbrain networks. Mov Disord. 2017;32:1006–15.

99. Gardner RC, Boxer AL, Trujillo A, et al. Intrinsic connectivity network disruption in progressive supranuclear palsy. Ann Neurol. 2013;73:603–16.

100. Bharti K, Bologna M, Upadhyay N, et al. Abnormal resting-state functional connectivity in progressive supranuclear palsy and Corticobasal syndrome. Front Neurol. 2017;8:248.

101. Upadhyay N, Suppa A, Piattella MC, et al. Functional disconnection of thalamic and cerebellar dentate nucleus networks in progressive supranuclear palsy and corticobasal syndrome. Parkinsonism Relat Disord. 2017;39:52–7.

102. Rosskopf J, Gorges M, Muller HP, et al. Hyperconnective and hypoconnective cortical and subcortical functional networks in multiple system atrophy. Parkinsonism Relat Disord. 2018;49:75–80.

103. Ren S, Zhang H, Zheng W, et al. Altered functional connectivity of Cerebello-cortical circuit in multiple system atrophy (cerebellar-type). Front Neurosci. 2018;12:996.

104. Yang H, Wang N, Luo X, et al. Altered functional connectivity of dentate nucleus in parkinsonian and cerebellar variants of multiple system atrophy. Brain Imaging Behav. 2019;13:1733–45.

105. Kawabata K, Hara K, Watanabe H, et al. Alterations in cognition-related Cerebello-cerebral networks in multiple system atrophy. Cerebellum. 2019;18:770–80.

106. Spinelli EG, Caso F, Agosta F, et al. A multimodal neuroimaging study of a case of crossed nonfluent/agrammatic primary progressive aphasia. J Neurol. 2015;262:2336–45.

107. Barkhof F, Fox NC, Bastos-Leite AJ, Scheltens P. Neuroimaging in dementia. Heidelberg: Springer; 2011.

Rapidly Progressive Dementias

5

Contents

5.1   Clinicopathological Findings

Rapidly progressive dementia (RPD) is a medical condition characterized by cognitive impairment typically developed over weeks to months [1]. Although there is not a standardized time frame to define a dementia as rapidly progressive, this term is usually referred to a condition that progresses from symptom onset to dementia in less than 1–2 years [1].

RPD may be caused by several nosological entities. In the largest available cohort of RPD patients [2], the majority of patients were found to be affected by a sporadic or genetic form of prion disease, while the remaining 38% were affected by a non-prion disease. Among patients with non-prion diseases, 39% were diagnosed with another neurodegenerative disease, 22% with autoimmune encephalitis and 4% with a disease of metabolic etiology [2]. According to the experience of two European tertiary care hospitals, the largest category of RPD was characterized by

© Springer Nature Switzerland AG 2021
M. Filippi, F. Agosta, *Imaging Dementia*,
https://doi.org/10.1007/978-3-030-66773-3_5

non-prion degenerative diseases, including Alzheimer's disease (AD) (17.6% and 14%), frontotemporal dementia (16.2% and 12%), and dementia with Lewy bodies (13.2% and 10%), whereas prion disease accounted for 13.2% and 30.6%, respectively [3, 4]. Of note, across different cohorts, a large proportion of cases is made of potentially treatable causes (i.e., immune-mediated disorders, neoplasms, infections, metabolic disorders) [1].

The following paragraphs will discuss the general diagnostic workup of RPD, focusing on neuroimaging findings in prion diseases, which represents the main single etiology. The discussion of other disorders that may present as RPD is referred to the specific chapters of the present text.

5.1.1   Diagnostic Workup

The first step in the evaluation of a patient with suspected RPD is the correct definition of the clinical history, in order to define the time course and the nature of symptoms at onset, which may orient toward a specific etiology [5, 6]. Routine blood test and urine analysis, to define the presence of common toxic-metabolic causes, should be performed [1]. The execution of an electroencephalographic (EEG) study is particularly useful if prion disease or encephalitis is suspected, or in case of seizures at disease onset or during the clinical progression [1]. Brain imaging is valuable to identify some peculiar features of specific diseases, as described in the following paragraphs, as well as to rule out several treatable etiologies (i.e., neoplasms, autoimmune disorders) or identify contraindications to the execution of a lumbar puncture. Regarding cerebrospinal fluid (CSF) analysis, pleocytosis or elevated IgG index or the presence of oligoclonal bands might indicate an autoimmune or inflammatory process, even though the presence of oligoclonal bands and alteration of the IgG index has been described also in relation to prion diseases [7]. Moreover, the evaluation of CSF neuronal injury biomarkers, such as 14-3-3 protein, and total and phosphorylated tau protein is recommended to confirm the history of a rapidly neurological condition and to direct the diagnosis [1].

For patients with an undiagnosed RPD after the initial workup, a body computed tomography (CT) scan with and without contrast should be performed to look for malignancies. If paraneoplastic antibodies are positive on serum or CSF evaluation, an aggressive cancer workup, including total body positron emission tomography (PET) with ^{18}F-fluorodeoxyglucose (FDG-PET), might be indicated [1].

Figure 5.1 shows a suggested algorithm for the initial evaluation of RPD [1].

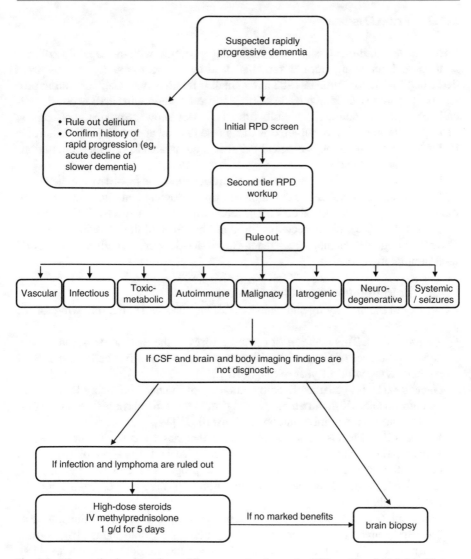

Fig. 5.1 Diagnostic algorithm for rapidly progressive dementia. *CSF* cerebrospinal fluid, *CT* computed tomography, *EEG* electroencephalogram, *MRI* magnetic resonance imaging, *PET* positron emission tomography. (Reproduced with permission from Geschwind MD. Rapidly Progressive Dementia. Continuum: Lifelong Learning in Neurology 2016; 22:510, https://journals.lww.com/continuum/pages/default.aspx)

5.1.2   Prion Diseases

Prions are small, infectious, protein-containing particles, with the capability of replicating and replacing normal proteins, leading to neurotoxicity. Prions were described for the first time in 1982 as "a small infectious pathogen containing protein but apparently lacking nucleic acid" [8]. The prion protein (PrP) is physiologically present in humans, although its function is not known. Some studies suggest its role in the activation of superoxide dismutase [9] and apoptosis [10]. Pathologic PrP is an isomer of the physiological PrP that accumulates in several brain regions and causes neurotoxicity.

Prion diseases are rare, transmissible, neurodegenerative disorders characterized by long incubation periods and common neuropathological features, with an inexorable progression after clinical onset. The most common prion disease is Creutzfeldt-Jakob disease (CJD), which accounts for more than 90% of the sporadic cases [11]. The remaining 10% includes Gerstmann-Straussler-Scheinker syndrome, kuru, and fatal familial insomnia.

5.1.2.1   Epidemiology and Classification

According to the underlying pathogenesis, CJD is classified in the following forms:

- *Sporadic CJD*. This is the most common form of the disease. Onset is usually between the ages of 50 and 70, with a median survival of 5 months and 85% of patients dying within 1 year of diagnosis [2].
- *Genetic CJD*. It is characterized by mutation of the gene encoding PrP, located on chromosome 20, with an autosomal dominant transmission. The most common mutations are point mutations and insertions [12].
- *Variant CJD*. This is an acquired disease that has been mostly described in younger adults with a mean age of 29 years [13, 14]. It has some differences in neuropathologic features, clinical onset, and progression compared to the sporadic form, representing the human infection with the agent of bovine spongiform encephalopathy [13, 14].
- *Iatrogenic CJD*. It is caused by medical procedures, such as the administration of cadaveric human pituitary hormones [15], dural graft transplants [16], corneal transplants [17], and use of contaminated neurosurgical instruments [18]. Iatrogenic CJD is believed to be controlled by current hygiene practices, and new incident cases are related to the very long incubation periods, with an estimated mean of 9–10 years [19], even though longer incubation time has been reported [20].

The vast majority of CJD cases are sporadic (85–95%), while 5–15% are due to the genetic form of CJD. Iatrogenic and variant forms of the disease account for less than 1% of the cases. The worldwide incidence is one per 1,000,000 individuals [21, 22]. Incidence is increased 30–100-fold in certain geographic regions due to clusters of genetic CJD [23].

Regarding the sporadic form of CJD, the PrP genotype allows a molecular classification in six subtypes, depending on the presence of a methionine (M) or a valine (V) at codon 129. This common polymorphism affects electrophoretic mobility of the protease-resistant core fragment, consequently influencing the risk of developing sporadic CJD and its clinical expression [24]. In fact, the presence of codon 129 MM is an established risk factor for sporadic CJD, and each molecular subtype is associated with a specific clinical presentation:

- MM1 and MV1 account for 70% of cases, determining the classic CJD phenotype, with advanced age onset, short duration of illness and rapidly progressive dementia and myoclonus [24].
- VV2 accounts for 10% of cases and presents with ataxia at onset as isolated feature, late dementia, and longer disease duration [25].
- MV2 accounts for approximately 10% of cases, characterized by ataxia, prominent psychiatric features, and dementia [26].
- MM2 is characterized by longer disease course and cerebellar signs and symptoms (4% of cases) [27].
- VV1 has a slower disease progression, dominated by dementia (1% of cases) [28].

5.1.2.2 Clinical Features
CJD is characterized by clinical heterogeneity, even though a common feature is the presence of rapid neuropsychiatric decline [29]. The most important clinical features of the disease include the following:

- Neuropsychiatric symptoms: these are the most frequent manifestations, in particular behavioral abnormalities, which are frequently associated with deficits of higher cortical function (i.e., aphasia, apraxia). As the disease progresses, dementia becomes dominant in most patients, with a rapid progression [30].
- Myoclonus: mainly exacerbated by startle, it is present in more than 90% of cases during the illness but may be absent at onset [31].
- Cerebellar and oculomotor manifestations: these occur in two-thirds of cases, including nystagmus and ataxia [31].
- Pyramidal involvement can be found in 40–80% of patients, including hyperreflexia, Babinski sign, and spasticity [31].
- Extrapyramidal signs including bradykinesia, dystonia, rigidity, and hypokinesia may also occur [31].

The mean age of onset is approximately 62 years, although cases in younger patients and those over 80 years old have been described [32–34]. End-stage sporadic CJD is typically characterized by akinetic mutism. During progression, myoclonus and spasticity become more frequent.

5.1.2.3 Diagnosis
CJD should be suspected in patients who present with RPD, particularly if accompanied by myoclonus and ataxia. Although neuropathologic examination remains

the gold standard for diagnosis, a diagnosis of probable CJD is often made with non-invasive testing, with appropriate clinical evaluation, laboratory and neuroimaging studies [35]. Table 5.1 shows the diagnostic criteria proposed by the Centers for Diseases Control and Prevention [36].

Neuroimaging, especially with magnetic resonance imaging (MRI), represents the most helpful instrumental test for the diagnosis of CJD (see sections below) [37]. EEG may also be a useful test, which might show the presence of a characteristic periodic synchronous bi- or triphasic periodic sharp wave complexes, observed

Table 5.1 Diagnostic criteria for CJD

1. Sporadic CJD
Definite
Diagnosed by standard neuropathological techniques; and/or immunocytochemically; and/or Western blot confirmed protease-resistant PrP; and/or presence of scrapie-associated fibrils.
Probable
Neuropsychiatric disorder plus positive RT-QuIC in cerebrospinal fluid (CSF) or other tissues
OR
Rapidly progressive dementia; **and** at least two of the following clinical features: 1. Myoclonus   2. Visual or cerebellar signs   3. Pyramidal/extrapyramidal signs   4. Akinetic mutism
AND a positive result on at least one of the following laboratory tests   1. A typical electroencephalogram (periodic sharp wave complexes) during an illness of any duration   2. A positive 14-3-3 CSF assay in patients with a disease duration of less than 2 years   3. High signal in caudate/putamen on MRI brain scan or at least two cortical regions (temporal, parietal, occipital) either on diffusion-weighted imaging or fluid-attenuated inversion recovery.
AND without routine investigations indicating an alternative diagnosis
Possible
Progressive dementia; **and** at least two out of the following four clinical features: 1. Myoclonus   2. Visual or cerebellar signs   3. Pyramidal/extrapyramidal signs   4. Akinetic mutism
AND the absence of a positive result for any of the four tests above that would classify a case as "probable"
AND duration of illness less than 2 years
AND without routine investigations indicating an alternative diagnosis.
2. Iatrogenic CJD
Progressive cerebellar syndrome in a recipient of human cadaveric-derived pituitary hormone; or sporadic CJD with a recognized exposure risk, e.g., antecedent neurosurgery with dura mater implantation.
3. Familial CJD
Definite or probable CJD **plus** definite or probable CJD in a first degree relative; and/or neuropsychiatric disorder **plus** disease-specific PrP gene mutation.

Reproduced from Diagnostic Criteria | Creutzfeldt-Jakob Disease, Classic (CJD) | Prion Disease | CDC. Available at: https://www.cdc.gov/prions/cjd/diagnostic-criteria.html.

in 67–95% of patients during the disease progression [38]. This finding represents a supportive but not definitive evidence of CJD, and even though it has high specificity, false-positive EEG results have been reported also in AD and vascular dementia cases [39]. Routine laboratory studies are typically normal in CJD.

CSF analysis should be considered as an adjunctive rather than a diagnostic test, due the mixed results regarding sensitivity and specificity of the detection of 14-3-3 and tau protein levels [40]. Regarding the detection of 14-3-3 protein in CSF, a negative test is not able to rule out the diagnosis, especially in cases of possible genetic and non-classical CJD [41]. On the other hand, a positive result can also occur in non-prion diseases, such as herpes simplex encephalitis and paraneoplastic diseases [42], although a positive finding increases the probability of CJD [43]. Some studies reported that the detection of elevated tau protein levels (>1150 pg/mL) has higher accuracy as a diagnostic test compared to 14-3-3, despite a significant number of false-negative and false-positive results [44]. Some studies have suggested the importance of evaluating the ratio of total tau to phosphorylated tau levels, with an elevated ratio as a marker with high specificity for CJD [45, 46]. The best diagnostic accuracy is reached using CSF real-time quacking-induced conversion (RT-QuIC), a diagnostic test which detects the prion seeding activity [47]. This technique has shown sensitivity and specificity ranging 87–91% and 98–100%, respectively [48].

5.2 Neuroimaging

5.2.1 Structural Neuroimaging

Structural neuroimaging has a key role in the evaluation of patients with RPD, particularly for the diagnosis of prion diseases. Although head CT is usually normal in CJD cases, it can be used to exclude alternative diagnoses. Serial CT scans over several months may show a rapid ventricular enlargement and progression of cortical atrophy, as atrophy might be sufficiently severe to be detected using CT in patients with advanced disease [49].

MRI has been demonstrated to be superior to CT in detecting abnormalities in patients with CJD [37], being the most accurate and useful neuroradiologic exam for excluding other potential causes of RPD and suggesting CJD as underlying etiology [37, 43]. The minimal recommended MRI protocol for the assessment of patients with RPD, especially if prion etiology is suspected, should include T2-weighted images, fluid-attenuated inversion recovery (FLAIR), T1-weighted images, and diffusion-weighted images (DWI) [50]. The administration of gadolinium contrast is not necessary, as it is not linked to specific MRI findings in prion diseases, but may be helpful to exclude other etiologies [50].

Currently, DWI is more useful for the diagnosis of prion disease than for any other dementia [51, 52], as hyperintensities of the cortical gyri (cortical ribboning), striatum (caudate and putamen), and/or thalamus on DWI scans are a common imaging feature in all forms of CJD (Fig. 5.2a, b, g), associated with correspondent

Fig. 5.2 Series of MRI scans of a sporadic Creutzfeldt-Jakob disease patient. DWI scan showing typical asymmetrical cortical signal hyperintensities (**a, b**). Hyperintensities in the same regions are shown also in FLAIR (**c, d**) and T2-weighted images (**e, f**). Hyperintensities in putamen and caudate nucleus head are evident on DWI scan (**g**). Hypointensities in areas with restricted diffusion are shown on the ADC map (**h**). Alterations are indicated by arrows

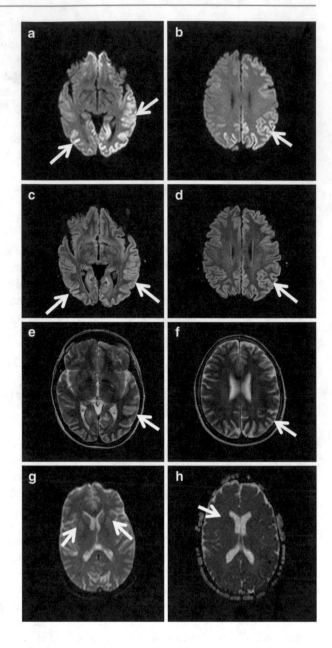

hypointensity on apparent diffusion coefficient (ADC) map (Fig. 5.2h) [51–56]. FLAIR/T2-weighted hyperintensities in the same areas may also be present, but they are less evident than DWI alterations in the vast majority of cases (Fig. 5.2c–f) [52, 55, 56]. Moreover, DWI alterations have been shown in the earliest phases of the disease, as these may be present even before the onset of clinical manifestations

[57, 58]. For the differentiation of CJD from non-prion RPD, MRI has shown sensitivities ranging between 83% and 94% [52, 59] with high inter-rater reliability [60], as compared to EEG (sensitivity 64% [39]) and CSF findings (sensitivity 92% [43]). The updated clinical diagnostic criteria of sporadic CJD include high signal abnormalities on DWI or FLAIR in the caudate nucleus and putamen or in at least two cortical regions as one of the supportive markers for the diagnosis of probable CJD, together with periodic sharp wave complexes on the EEG and 14-3-3 protein detection in the CSF [55].

The neuroradiological picture, mainly related to DWI signal alterations, reflects neuronal vacuolation and reactive astrogliosis [61] caused by the deposition of PrP [62], with subsequent reduced diffusion of water molecules. Disease progression is accompanied by a consistent increase in the extent and degree of signal intensity on T2-weighted images and DWI, mainly in subcortical gray matter regions [63]. Higher intensity correlates with increasing disease duration and degree of spongiform degeneration [63], although, in some cases at a later disease stage, these intensity abnormalities may decrease or disappear on DWI studies [57]. This observation is suggested to be related to neuronal loss and brain atrophy progression [63].

In sporadic CJD, the most common patterns of DWI hyperintensities are neocortical, limbic, and subcortical (54–68% of cases), and neocortical and limbic (24–27% of cases) [51, 52]. There is no neocortical involvement in 5–11% of patients with sporadic CJD [51, 52]. Cortical areas most commonly involved are the cingulate gyrus, superior and middle frontal gyrus, insula, precuneus, angular gyrus, and parahippocampal gyrus, with a relative sparing of the precentral gyrus [52]. Striatal hyperintensity almost always shows an anterior-to-posterior gradient, with prevalent involvement of the caudate and relative sparing of the posterior putamen. Thalamic alterations on DWI are usually bilateral, involving the dorsomedian and posterior (pulvinar) regions [52]. The DWI hyperintensity in subcortical regions almost invariably corresponds to a hypointensity on the apparent diffusion coefficient map, confirming a pattern of restricted diffusion [52].

There are also unusual recognizable patterns that might be useful for the differential diagnostic workup. A confluent hyperintensity in the posterior thalami (pulvinar) and a confluent hyperintensity in the dorsomedial thalami on T2-weighted, FLAIR, and DWI sequences are named, respectively, "pulvinar sign" and "double hockey-stick sign" (Fig. 5.3). These signs are the most indicative neuroimaging markers for variant CJD [64]. Thalamic involvement is not pathognomonic for variant CJD, as it has been reported also in cases of sporadic prion disease [65], although these presentations are more commonly characterized by relative sparing of the thalamus and more severe striatal and neocortical involvement [66]. An additional unusual finding associated with sporadic CJD is the hyperintensity in the globus pallidus on T1-weighted images, in the absence of DWI abnormalities [66], caused by a heavy deposition of PrP in this area [67].

Intriguingly, despite the intense pathologic involvement of the cerebellum and the high prevalence of clinically evident cerebellar signs, CJD patients typically do

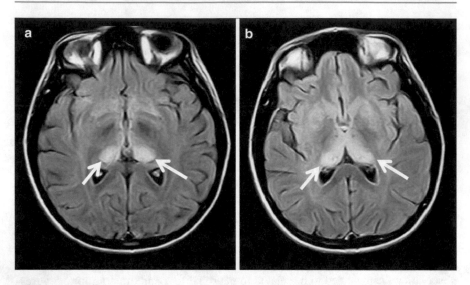

Fig. 5.3 FLAIR scans showing (**a**) the "pulvinar sign," as a confluent hyperintensity in the posterior thalami, and (**b**) symmetrical pulvinar and dorsomedial thalamic nuclear hyperintensity, giving a characteristic "double hockey-stick" appearance. Alterations are indicated by arrows. (Reproduced with permission from Collie DA, Summers DM, Sellar RJ, et al. Diagnosing variant Creutzfeldt-Jakob disease with the pulvinar sign: MR imaging findings in 86 neuropathologically confirmed cases. AJNR Am J Neuroradiol 2003; 24:1560–1569)

not display MRI cerebellar alterations [51, 68]. Cerebellar involvement can be suggested by atrophy and elevated diffusivity, identifiable mainly on ADC maps, but poorly visualized in non-quantitative DWI [68]. Only a few reports described DWI hyperintensities in this region [69].

According to the molecular classification of CJD, characteristic lesion patterns on DWI and T2WI/FLAIR studies have been described for each molecular subtype: basal ganglia hyperintensities occur most frequently in MV2, VV2, and MM1 subtypes, whereas cortical signal alterations are most common in VV1, MM2, and MV1 subtypes (Fig. 5.4) [70]. Thalamic involvement occurs most frequently in VV2 and MV2 molecular subtypes (Fig. 5.4) [70].

In Table 5.2, a summary of typical imaging features in CJD is reported.

5.2.2   Molecular Imaging

Functional neuroimaging techniques, such as PET and single photon emission computed tomography (SPECT), are sensitive in early stages of prion disease as they can show diminished lobar metabolism [71] even before morphologic MRI and CT abnormalities are detectable [72]. Despite the higher sensitivity of nuclear medicine imaging for early diagnosis, these techniques are not routinely included in the diagnostic workup, due to their low specificity, related to the great variability of hypoperfused/hypometabolic patterns [73].

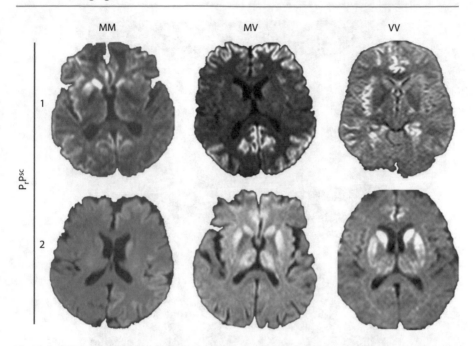

Fig. 5.4 DWI of six sporadic Creutzfeldt-Jakob disease patients with various molecular subtypes. Basal ganglia hyperintensities occur most frequently in MV2, VV2, and MM1 subtypes, whereas cortical signal alterations are most common in VV1, MM2, and MV1 subtypes. Thalamic involvement occurs most frequently in VV2 and MV2 molecular subtypes. (Reproduced from Meissner B, Kallenberg K, Sanchez-Juan P, et al. MRI lesion profiles in sporadic Creutzfeldt-Jakob disease. Neurology 2009; 72:1994–2001, https://n.neurology.org/)

Table 5.2 Summary of typical imaging appearances in CJD

Region	Feature	Sequences
Cerebral cortex	Focal or diffuse, symmetric or asymmetric involvement. Prerolandic usually spared	FLAIR and mainly DWI/ADC. Signal intensity abnormality may fluctuate
Basal ganglia	Symmetric or asymmetric involvement, particularly of caudate and putamen	FLAIR and mainly DWI/ADC. Increase in both extent and degree of signal intensity abnormality with progression
Cerebellum	Atrophy	T1-weighted images

Reproduced with permission from Fragoso DC, Gonçalves Filho AL, Pacheco FT, Barros BR, Aguiar Littig I, Nunes RH, Maia Júnior AC, da Rocha AJ. Imaging of Creutzfeldt-Jakob Disease: Imaging Patterns and Their Differential Diagnosis. RadioGraphics 2017; 37: 234–257
Abbreviations: *ADC* apparent diffusion coefficient, *DWI* diffusion-weighted imaging, *FLAIR* fluid-attenuated inversion recovery

Using FDG-PET, cortical and subcortical hypometabolism is commonly observed (Fig. 5.5) [74]. Even though this pattern shows an important inter-subject variability, the frontal cortex, thalamus, and caudate are most frequently affected [74]. Considering the cortical involvement, it is usually lateralized and located in

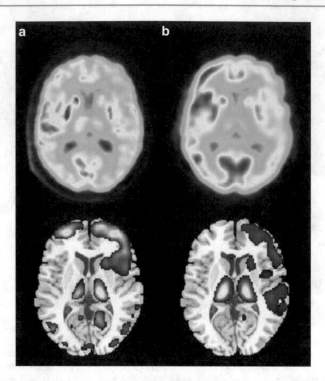

Fig. 5.5 FDG-PET image and corresponding hypometabolic map in sporadic and variant Creutzfeldt-Jakob disease (CJD). (**a**) Sporadic CJD patient shows bilateral thalamic hypometabolism and frontal impairment. (**b**) The patient with variant CJD presents a highly significant thalamic depletion with hypometabolism in the left frontal and temporal cortex. (Reprinted by permission from Springer Nature: Springer-Verlag Berlin Heidelberg, Eur J Nucl Med Mol Imaging, Metabolic patterns in prion diseases: an FDG-PET voxel-based analysis, Prieto E, Domínguez-Prado I, Riverol M, et al. Copyright, 2015)

the medial and lateral parts of the frontal and parietal cortex [74, 75]. Moreover, mirroring the variability of CJD clinical picture, also FDG-PET imaging findings, may include, in addition to the typical lateral frontal and mesial parietal hypometabolism, involvement of the pons and middle cerebellar peduncles in patients with ataxia, as well as the occipital cortex in patients with visual clinical signs [76]. The knowledge regarding PET hypometabolic patterns is still limited due the lack of studies assessing large cohorts of patients.

In consideration of FDG-PET utility in the clinical setting, this technique might be helpful in the diagnosis of CJD in case of lack of complete workup, such as in the presence of contraindications to MRI scan (e.g., a pace-maker) or lumbar puncture. In general, the presence of MRI abnormalities, associated with typical EEG and CSF findings, make FDG-PET non-essential for the diagnosis of CJD [77].

An important characteristic of PET studies is the possibility of using different tracers. Amyloid tracers are widely used in the research field in several neurodegenerative disease, although regarding CJD these tracers showed controversial results, according to the different tracers used [78, 79]. Even though evidence is still limited, it has been suggested that amyloid tracers may not be entirely selective and may bind to other proteins deposited, such as PrP. According to this observation, a study showed that the uptake of ^{18}F-florbetaben, but not FDG, correlated with the amount of pathological PrP in the pathological examination of the brain [80].

5.2.3 Advanced MRI Techniques

Even though conventional structural MRI findings are mostly related to gray matter abnormalities, there is histopathologic evidence that white matter damage occurs, with reactive diffuse astrocytic gliosis, activated microglia, vacuolation, and rare PrP deposition [81]. Studies based on diffusion tensor imaging (DTI) showed a widespread white matter involvement in sporadic CJD, as the result of microstructural abnormalities, which are invisible with conventional techniques (Fig. 5.6) [81, 82]. These are characterized mainly by a diffuse reduction of mean diffusivity (MD) and a regional decrease of fractional anisotropy (FA) in frontal and cingulate

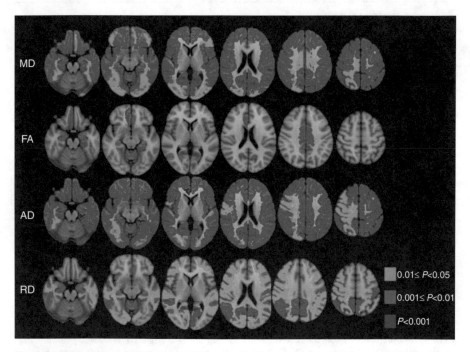

Fig. 5.6 Cross-sectional white matter DTI analysis. Figure shows reduced mean diffusivity, fractional anisotropy, axial diffusivity, and/or radial diffusivity in sporadic Creutzfeldt-Jakob disease patients compared with controls. Color scale shows *P*-values of significance. *AD* axial diffusivity, *FA* fractional anisotropy, *MD* mean diffusivity, *RD* radial diffusivity. (Reproduced from Caverzasi E, Mandelli ML, DeArmond SJ, et al. White matter involvement in sporadic Creutzfeldt-Jakob disease. Brain 2014; 137:3339–3354, by permission of Oxford University Press)

cortices [81, 82]. Significant decreases in mean, axial, and radial diffusivity were also observed in the deep nuclei, such as thalamus, putamen, and globus pallidus, accompanied by a reduction in fractional anisotropy in several brain regions, such as frontal, temporal, parietal and occipital lobes, corpus callosum, and cerebellum [83]. The longitudinal evolution of MD values showed an interesting pattern: during the disease course the MD change is not unidirectional as an initial rapid decrease is followed by a slower reduction. The decrease in MD, characteristic of the first phases of the disease, might arrest and, in some cases, reverse with a progressive increase, called "relative normalization," up to a clearly abnormal increased MD [84]. This biphasic pattern of MD longitudinal evolution is explained by an initial prominent deposition of PrP and microvacuolation that lead to the typical spongi-form pathologic alteration with consequently reduced diffusion of water molecules in tissues and, accordingly, decreased MD. As the disease progresses, the prominent atrophy due to neuronal loss and fiber disruption causes a progressive increase in diffusion of water molecules, with subsequent increase of MD [81, 85]. A strong relationship between changes in clinical functional impairment and MD alterations has been described [84].

5.3   Clinical Case #1

A 70-year-old man was completely independent in his activities of daily living and instrumental activities of daily living until 6 months earlier, when his family noticed the development of cognitive decline with memory issues, word-finding difficulty, associated with unsteady gait. The patient was conducted to the emergency depart-ment due to the worsening of the described clinical picture, with confusion devel-oped over 2 weeks.

His past medical history was significant for coronary artery disease and hyper-tension. General physical examination was unremarkable. Neurological examina-tion revealed expressive aphasia and ideomotor apraxia, associated to myoclonus and lower limb hyperreflexia.

His routine blood exams, including white blood cell count, hemoglobin, plate-lets, electrolytes, and vitamins, were within normal limits. Syphilis and HIV serolo-gies were both negative, as was the antinuclear antibodies. MRI demonstrated ventricular enlargement that was prominent for age associated with asymmetrical hyperintensities on FLAIR (Fig. 5.7a, b) and DWI scans (Fig. 5.7c, d), located mainly in basal ganglia and cerebral hemispheric cortex. EEG was abnormal but nonspecific, without epileptic activity. CSF showed a normal nucleated cell count, normal glucose, slightly elevated proteins, no oligoclonal bands. On the other hand, CSF showed greatly increased levels of tau and 14-3-3 protein. Paraneoplastic anti-bodies (anti-Hu, Ri, Yo, Ma2, Cv2, and amphiphysin) were negative. End-point quaking-induced conversion (EP-QuIC) was performed and resulted positive. The diagnostic criteria for possible sporadic CJD were fulfilled.

In the subsequent 6 weeks he developed mutism, and passed away 8 weeks after his initial presentation. The postmortem autopsy was consistent with sporadic CJD.

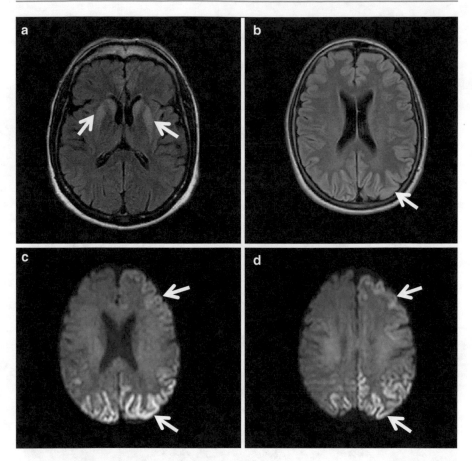

Fig. 5.7 FLAIR (**a, b**) and DWI (**c, d**) MR scans showing asymmetrical cortical and basal ganglia hyperintensities in clinical case #1 (sporadic Creutzfeldt-Jakob disease). Alterations are indicated by arrows

5.4   Clinical Case #2

A 56-year-old man presented to the emergency department with a memory decline steadily worsening over a 2-week period, with prominent involvement of antero-grade memory. The neurological examination did not show relevant findings apart from the cognitive impairment. The scores at the Mini-Mental State Examination (MMSE) and Montreal Cognitive Assessment (MoCA) were respectively 19/30 and 15/30. No epileptic seizures occurred. Patient's previous medical history was nega-tive for relevant medical conditions.

CSF analysis showed mildly elevated leukocyte (19/u) and normal protein and glucose levels (44 mg/dL, normal range 20–40 mg/dL). At the same time, the serum tests of sodium, chloride, and blood glucose were 126.1, 94.2, and 7.26 mmol/L, respectively. EEG and initial brain MRI were normal. The MRI scan performed 2

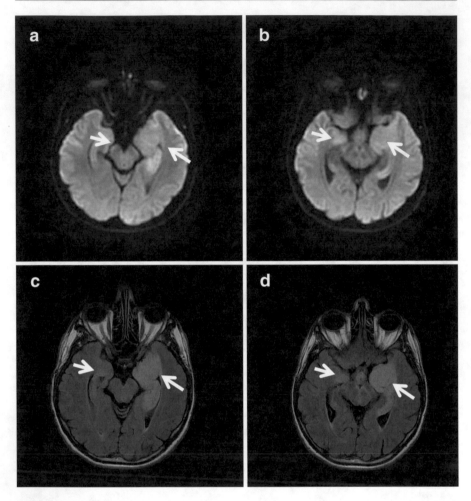

Fig. 5.8 DWI (**a, b**) and FLAIR (**c, d**) MR scans of an anti-LGI1 autoimmune encephalitis patient (clinical case #2). Asymmetrical hyperintensities in bilateral mesial temporal lobes on FLAIR and DWI images are evident (arrows), with a prominent involvement of the left temporal lobe

weeks later showed asymmetrical hyperintensities in bilateral mesial temporal lobes on DWI (Fig. 5.8a, b) and FLAIR (Fig. 5.8c, d) images. Chest and abdomen contrast enhanced computed tomography and total body FDG-PET showed no signs of tumor. LGI1 antibodies were positive both in the serum and CSF. Blood tumor markers and other paraneoplastic neuronal antibodies were all unremarkable.

He was diagnosed with anti-LGI1 autoimmune encephalitis and treated with intravenous immunoglobulin and later with oral prednisone for 6 months. Fifteen days after his admission, he was discharged from hospital with mild memory impairment.

See Book Introduction for an overview of other treatable causes of dementia.

References

1. Geschwind MD. Rapidly progressive dementia. Continuum Lifelong Learn Neurol. 2016;22:510–37.
2. Geschwind MD, Shu H, Haman A, Sejvar JJ, Miller BL. Rapidly progressive dementia. Ann Neurol. 2008;64:97.
3. Papageorgiou SG, Kontaxis T, Bonakis A, et al. Rapidly progressive dementia: causes found in a Greek tertiary referral center in Athens. Alzheimer Dis Assoc Disord. 2009;23:337–46.
4. Sala I, Marquié M, Sánchez-Saudinós MB, et al. Rapidly progressive dementia: experience in a tertiary care medical center. Alzheimer Dis Assoc Disord. 2012;26:267–71.
5. Lindau M, Almkvist O, Kushi J, et al. First symptoms—frontotemporal dementia versus Alzheimer's disease. Dement Geriatr Cogn Disord. 2000;11:286–93.
6. Claassen DO, Josephs KA, Ahlskog JE, et al. REM sleep behavior disorder preceding other aspects of synucleinopathies by up to half a century. Neurology. 2010;75:494–9.
7. Geschwind MD. Prion diseases. Continuum (Minneap Minn). 2015;21:1612–38.
8. Prusiner SB. Novel proteinaceous infectious particles cause scrapie. Science. 1982;216:136–44.
9. Sakudo A, Lee DC, Nishimura T, et al. Octapeptide repeat region and N-terminal half of hydrophobic region of prion protein (PrP) mediate PrP-dependent activation of superoxide dismutase. Biochem Biophys Res Commun. 2005;326:600–6.
10. Solforosi L, Criado JR, McGavern DB, et al. Cross-linking cellular prion protein triggers neuronal apoptosis in vivo. Science. 2004;303:1514–6.
11. Puoti G, Bizzi A, Forloni G, et al. Sporadic human prion diseases: molecular insights and diagnosis. Lancet Neurol. 2012;11:618–28.
12. Knight RS, Will RG. Prion diseases. J Neurol Neurosurg Psychiatry. 2004;75(Suppl 1):i36–42.
13. Will RG, Ironside JW, Zeidler M, et al. A new variant of Creutzfeldt-Jakob disease in the UK. Lancet. 1996;347:921–5.
14. Collinge J, Rossor M. A new variant of prion disease. Lancet. 1996;347:916–7.
15. Lewis AM, Yu M, DeArmond SJ, et al. Human growth hormone–related iatrogenic Creutzfeldt-Jakob disease with abnormal imaging. Arch Neurol. 2006;63:288.
16. Hamaguchi T, Sakai K, Noguchi-Shinohara M, et al. Insight into the frequent occurrence of dura mater graft-associated Creutzfeldt-Jakob disease in Japan. J Neurol Neurosurg Psychiatry. 2013;84:1171–5.
17. Allan B, Tuft S. Transmission of Creutzfeldt-Jakob disease in corneal grafts. BMJ. 1997;315:1553–4.
18. Johnson RT, Gibbs CJ. Creutzfeldt–Jakob disease and related transmissible spongiform encephalopathies. N Engl J Med. 1998;339:1994–2004.
19. Heath CA. Dura mater-associated Creutzfeldt-Jakob disease: experience from surveillance in the UK. J Neurol Neurosurg Psychiatry. 2006;77:880–2.
20. Furtner M, Gelpi E, Kiechl S, et al. Iatrogenic Creutzfeldt Jakob disease 22 years after human growth hormone therapy: clinical and radiological features. J Neurol Neurosurg Psychiatry. 2008;79:229–31.
21. Masters CL, Harris JO, Gajdusek DC, et al. Creutzfeldt-Jakob disease: patterns of worldwide occurrence and the significance of familial and sporadic clustering. Ann Neurol. 1979;5:177–88.
22. Ladogana A, Puopolo M, Croes EA, et al. Mortality from Creutzfeldt-Jakob disease and related disorders in Europe, Australia, and Canada. Neurology. 2005;64:1586–91.
23. Ladogana A, Puopolo M, Poleggi A, et al. High incidence of genetic human transmissible spongiform encephalopathies in Italy. Neurology. 2005;64:1592–7.
24. Parchi P, Giese A, Capellari S, et al. Classification of sporadic Creutzfeldt-Jakob disease based on molecular and phenotypic analysis of 300 subjects. Ann Neurol. 1999;46:224–33.
25. Cooper SA, Murray KL, Heath CA, Will RG, Knight RSG. Sporadic Creutzfeldt-Jakob disease with cerebellar ataxia at onset in the UK. J Neurol Neurosurg Psychiatry. 2006;77:1273–5.
26. Krasnianski A. Clinical findings and diagnostic tests in the MV2 subtype of sporadic CJD. Brain. 2006;129:2288–96.

27. Krasnianski A, Meissner B, Schulz-Schaeffer W, et al. Clinical features and diagnosis of the MM2 cortical subtype of sporadic Creutzfeldt-Jakob disease. Arch Neurol. 2006;63:876.
28. Meissner B, Westner IM, Kallenberg K, et al. Sporadic Creutzfeldt-Jakob disease: clinical and diagnostic characteristics of the rare VV1 type. Neurology. 2005;65:1544–50.
29. Haywood AM. Transmissible spongiform encephalopathies. N Engl J Med. 1997;337:1821–8.
30. Krasnianski A, Bohling GT, Heinemann U, et al. Neuropsychological symptoms in sporadic Creutzfeldt-Jakob disease patients in Germany. J Alzheimers Dis. 2017;59:329–37.
31. Rabinovici GD, Wang PN, Levin J, et al. First symptom in sporadic Creutzfeldt-Jakob disease. Neurology. 2006;66:286–7.
32. Monreal J, Collins GH, Masters CL, et al. Creutzfeldt-Jakob disease in an adolescent. J Neurol Sci. 1981;52:341–50.
33. de Silva R, Findlay C, Awad I, et al. Creutzfeldt-Jakob disease in the elderly. Postgrad Med J. 1997;73:557–9.
34. Johnson RT, Gonzalez RG, Frosch MP. Case records of the Massachusetts General Hospital. Case 27-2005. An 80-year-old man with fatigue, unsteady gait, and confusion. N Engl J Med. 2005;353:1042–50.
35. Brandel JP, Delasnerie-Lauprêtre N, Laplanche JL, Hauw JJ, Alpérovitch A. Diagnosis of Creutzfeldt-Jakob disease: effect of clinical criteria on incidence estimates. Neurology. 2000;54:1095–9.
36. Diagnostic criteria | Creutzfeldt-Jakob disease, classic (CJD) | Prion disease | CDC, 2019.
37. Macfarlane RG, Wroe SJ, Collinge J, Yousry TA, Jager HR. Neuroimaging findings in human prion disease. J Neurol Neurosurg Psychiatry. 2006;78:664–70.
38. Steinhoff BJ, Racker S, Herrendorf G, et al. Accuracy and reliability of periodic sharp wave complexes in Creutzfeldt-Jakob disease. Arch Neurol. 1996;53:162–6.
39. Steinhoff BJ, Zerr I, Glatting M, et al. Diagnostic value of periodic complexes in Creutzfeldt-Jakob disease. Ann Neurol. 2004;56:702–8.
40. Collins SJ. Determinants of diagnostic investigation sensitivities across the clinical spectrum of sporadic Creutzfeldt-Jakob disease. Brain. 2006;129:2278–87.
41. Sanchez-Juan P, Green A, Ladogana A, et al. CSF tests in the differential diagnosis of Creutzfeldt-Jakob disease. Neurology. 2006;67:637–43.
42. Chapman T, McKeel DW, Morris JC. Misleading results with the 14-3-3 assay for the diagnosis of Creutzfeldt-Jakob disease. Neurology. 2000;55:1396–8.
43. Muayqil T, Gronseth G, Camicioli R. Evidence-based guideline: diagnostic accuracy of CSF 14-3-3 protein in sporadic Creutzfeldt-Jakob disease: report of the guideline development subcommittee of the American Academy of Neurology. Neurology. 2012;79:1499–506.
44. Hamlin C, Puoti G, Berri S, et al. A comparison of tau and 14-3-3 protein in the diagnosis of Creutzfeldt-Jakob disease. Neurology. 2012;79:547–52.
45. Otto M, Wiltfang J, Cepek L, et al. Tau protein and 14-3-3 protein in the differential diagnosis of Creutzfeldt-Jakob disease. Neurology. 2002;58:192–7.
46. Zanusso G, Fiorini M, Farinazzo A, et al. Phosphorylated 14-3-3zeta protein in the CSF of neuroleptic-treated patients. Neurology. 2005;64:1618–20.
47. Green AJE, Zanusso G. Prion protein amplification techniques. In: Human prion diseases. Amsterdam: Elsevier; 2018. p. 357–70.
48. McGuire LI, Peden AH, Orrú CD, et al. Real time quaking-induced conversion analysis of cerebrospinal fluid in sporadic Creutzfeldt-Jakob disease. Ann Neurol. 2012;72:278–85.
49. Hayashi R, Hanyu N, Kuwabara T, Moriyama S. Serial computed tomographic and electroencephalographic studies in Creutzfeldt-Jakob disease. Acta Neurol Scand. 2009;85:161–5.
50. Collie DA, Sellar RJ, Zeidler M, et al. MRI of Creutzfeldt–Jakob disease: imaging features and recommended MRI protocol. Clin Radiol. 2001;56:726–39.
51. Young GS, Geschwind MD, Fischbein NJ, et al. Diffusion-weighted and fluid-attenuated inversion recovery imaging in Creutzfeldt-Jakob disease: high sensitivity and specificity for diagnosis. AJNR Am J Neuroradiol. 2005;26:1551–62.
52. Vitali P, Maccagnano E, Caverzasi E, et al. Diffusion-weighted MRI hyperintensity patterns differentiate CJD from other rapid dementias. Neurology. 2011;76:1711–9.

53. Murata T, Shiga Y, Higano S, Takahashi S, Mugikura S. Conspicuity and evolution of lesions in Creutzfeldt-Jakob disease at diffusion-weighted imaging. AJNR Am J Neuroradiol. 2002;23:1164–72.

54. Shiga Y, Miyazawa K, Sato S, et al. Diffusion-weighted MRI abnormalities as an early diagnostic marker for Creutzfeldt-Jakob disease. Neurology. 2004;63:443–9.

55. Zerr I, Kallenberg K, Summers DM, et al. Updated clinical diagnostic criteria for sporadic Creutzfeldt-Jakob disease. Brain. 2009;132:2659–68.

56. Fujita K, Harada M, Sasaki M, et al. Multicentre multiobserver study of diffusion-weighted and fluid-attenuated inversion recovery MRI for the diagnosis of sporadic Creutzfeldt-Jakob disease: a reliability and agreement study. BMJ Open. 2012;2:e000649.

57. Ukisu R, Kushihashi T, Kitanosono T, et al. Serial diffusion-weighted MRI of Creutzfeldt-Jakob disease. Am J Roentgenol. 2005;184:560–6.

58. Alvarez FJ, Bisbe J, Bisbe V, Davalos A. Magnetic resonance imaging findings in pre-clinical Creutzfeldt-Jakob disease. Int J Neurosci. 2005;115:1219–25.

59. Zeidler M, Green A. Advances in diagnosing Creutzfeldt-Jakob disease with MRI and CSF 14-3-3 protein analysis. Neurology. 2004;63:410–1.

60. Tschampa HJ, Kallenberg K, Urbach H, et al. MRI in the diagnosis of sporadic Creutzfeldt–Jakob disease: a study on inter-observer agreement. Brain. 2005;128:2026–33.

61. Falcone S, Quencer RM, Bowen B, Bruce JH, Naidich TP. Creutzfeldt-Jakob disease: focal symmetrical cortical involvement demonstrated by MR imaging. AJNR Am J Neuroradiol. 1992;13:403–6.

62. Na DL, Suh CK, Choi SH, et al. Diffusion-weighted magnetic resonance imaging in probable Creutzfeldt-Jakob disease: a clinical-anatomic correlation. Arch Neurol. 1999;56:951–7.

63. Fragoso DC, Gonçalves Filho AL, Pacheco FT, et al. Imaging of Creutzfeldt-Jakob disease: imaging patterns and their differential diagnosis. Radiographics. 2017;37:234–57.

64. Collie DA, Summers DM, Sellar RJ, et al. Diagnosing variant Creutzfeldt-Jakob disease with the pulvinar sign: MR imaging findings in 86 neuropathologically confirmed cases. AJNR Am J Neuroradiol. 2003;24:1560–9.

65. Petzold GC, Westner I, Bohner G, et al. False-positive pulvinar sign on MRI in sporadic Creutzfeldt-Jakob disease. Neurology. 2004;62:1235–6.

66. Kallenberg K, Schulz-Schaeffer WJ, Jastrow U, et al. Creutzfeldt-Jakob disease: comparative analysis of MR imaging sequences. AJNR Am J Neuroradiol. 2006;27:1459–62.

67. de Priester JA, Jansen GH, de Kruijk JR, Wilmink JT. New MRI findings in Creutzfeldt-Jakob disease: high signal in the globus pallidus on T1-weighted images. Neuroradiology. 1999;41:265–8.

68. Cohen OS, Hoffmann C, Lee H, et al. MRI detection of the cerebellar syndrome in Creutzfeldt-Jakob disease. Cerebellum. 2009;8:373–81.

69. Poon MA, Stuckey S, Storey E. MRI evidence of cerebellar and hippocampal involvement in Creutzfeldt-Jakob disease. Neuroradiology. 2001;43:746–9.

70. Meissner B, Kallenberg K, Sanchez-Juan P, et al. MRI lesion profiles in sporadic Creutzfeldt-Jakob disease. Neurology. 2009;72:1994–2001.

71. Henkel K, Zerr I, Hertel A, et al. Positron emission tomography with [(18)F]FDG in the diagnosis of Creutzfeldt-Jakob disease (CJD). J Neurol. 2002;249:699–705.

72. Xing XW, Zhang JT, Zhu F, et al. Comparison of diffusion-weighted MRI with 18F-fluorodeoxyglucose-positron emission tomography/CT and electroencephalography in sporadic Creutzfeldt-Jakob disease. J Clin Neurosci. 2012;19:1354–7.

73. Fragoso DC, Gonçalves Filho AL, Pacheco FT, Barros BR, Aguiar Littig I, Nunes RH, Maia Júnior AC, da Rocha AJ. Imaging of Creutzfeldt-Jakob disease: imaging patterns and their differential diagnosis. Radiographics. 2017;37:234–57.

74. Prieto E, Domínguez-Prado I, Riverol M, et al. Metabolic patterns in prion diseases: an FDG PET voxel-based analysis. Eur J Nucl Med Mol Imaging. 2015;42:1522–9.

75. Kim EJ, Cho SS, Jeong BH, et al. Glucose metabolism in sporadic Creutzfeldt-Jakob disease: a statistical parametric mapping analysis of (18) F-FDG PET. Eur J Neurol. 2012;19:488–93.

76. Renard D, Vandenberghe R, Collombier L, et al. Glucose metabolism in nine patients with probable sporadic Creutzfeldt-Jakob disease: FDG-PET study using SPM and individual patient analysis. J Neurol. 2013;260:3055–64.
77. Renard D, Castelnovo G, Collombier L, Thouvenot E, Boudousq V. FDG-PET in Creutzfeldt-Jakob disease: analysis of clinical-PET correlation. Prion. 2017;11:440–53.
78. Villemagne VL, McLean CA, Reardon K, et al. 11C-PiB PET studies in typical sporadic Creutzfeldt-Jakob disease. J Neurol Neurosurg Psychiatry. 2009;80:998–1001.
79. Okamura N, Shiga Y, Furumoto S, et al. In vivo detection of prion amyloid plaques using [(11)C]BF-227 PET. Eur J Nucl Med Mol Imaging. 2010;37:934–41.
80. Matías-Guiu JA, Guerrero-Márquez C, Cabrera-Martín MN, et al. Amyloid- and FDG-PET in sporadic Creutzfeldt-Jakob disease: correlation with pathological prion protein in neuropathology. Prion. 2017;11:205–13.
81. Caverzasi E, Mandelli ML, DeArmond SJ, et al. White matter involvement in sporadic Creutzfeldt-Jakob disease. Brain. 2014;137:3339–54.
82. Liu W, Wong A, Au L, et al. Influence of amyloid-beta on cognitive decline after stroke/transient ischemic attack: three-year longitudinal study. Stroke. 2015;46:3074–80.
83. Grau-Rivera O, Calvo A, Bargallo N, et al. Quantitative magnetic resonance abnormalities in Creutzfeldt-Jakob disease and fatal insomnia. J Alzheimers Dis. 2017;55:431–43.
84. Caverzasi E, Henry RG, Vitali P, et al. Application of quantitative DTI metrics in sporadic CJD. Neuroimage Clin. 2014;4:426–35.
85. Tschampa HJ, Kallenberg K, Kretzschmar HA, et al. Pattern of cortical changes in sporadic Creutzfeldt-Jakob disease. AJNR Am J Neuroradiol. 2007;28:1114–8.

Printed in the United States
by Baker & Taylor Publisher Services